AF781547

MULTIPLE SCLEROSIS RESEARCH PROGRESS

MULTIPLE SCLEROSIS RESEARCH PROGRESS

HANNA SCHWARZ AND LENA WALTER
EDITORS

Nova Science Publishers, Inc.
New York

Copyright © 2008 by Nova Science Publishers, Inc.

All rights reserved. No part of this book may be reproduced, stored in a retrieval system or transmitted in any form or by any means: electronic, electrostatic, magnetic, tape, mechanical photocopying, recording or otherwise without the written permission of the Publisher.

For permission to use material from this book please contact us:
Telephone 631-231-7269; Fax 631-231-8175
Web Site: http://www.novapublishers.com

NOTICE TO THE READER

The Publisher has taken reasonable care in the preparation of this book, but makes no expressed or implied warranty of any kind and assumes no responsibility for any errors or omissions. No liability is assumed for incidental or consequential damages in connection with or arising out of information contained in this book. The Publisher shall not be liable for any special, consequential, or exemplary damages resulting, in whole or in part, from the readers' use of, or reliance upon, this material.

Independent verification should be sought for any data, advice or recommendations contained in this book. In addition, no responsibility is assumed by the publisher for any injury and/or damage to persons or property arising from any methods, products, instructions, ideas or otherwise contained in this publication.

This publication is designed to provide accurate and authoritative information with regard to the subject matter covered herein. It is sold with the clear understanding that the Publisher is not engaged in rendering legal or any other professional services. If legal or any other expert assistance is required, the services of a competent person should be sought. FROM A DECLARATION OF PARTICIPANTS JOINTLY ADOPTED BY A COMMITTEE OF THE AMERICAN BAR ASSOCIATION AND A COMMITTEE OF PUBLISHERS.

LIBRARY OF CONGRESS CATALOGING-IN-PUBLICATION DATA

Multiple sclerosis research progress / Hanna Schwarz and Lena Walter (editors).
p. ; cm.
Includes bibliographical references and index.
ISBN 978-1-60456-570-6 (hardcover)
1. Multiple sclerosis. I. Schwarz, Hanna, 1958- II. Walter, Lena.
[DNLM: 1. Multiple Sclerosis. WL 360 M96192 2008]
RC377.M8675 2008
616.8'34--dc22
2008013217

Published by Nova Science Publishers, Inc. ✦ New York

CONTENTS

PREFACE

Multiple sclerosis (MS) is a life-long chronic disease diagnosed primarily in young adults. During an MS attack, inflammation occurs in areas of the white matter of the central nervous system (nerve fibers that are the site of MS lesions) in random patches called plaques. This process is followed by destruction of myelin, which insulates nerve cell fibers in the brain and spinal cord. Myelin facilitates the smooth, high-speed transmission of electrochemical messages between the brain, the spinal cord, and the rest of the body. The initial symptom of MS is often blurred or double vision, red-green color distortion, or even blindness in one eye. Most MS patients experience muscle weakness in their extremities and difficulty with coordination and balance. Most people with MS also exhibit paresthesias, transitory abnormal sensory feeling such as numbness or "pins and needles." Some may experience pain or loss of feeling. About half of people with MS experience cognitive impairments such as difficulties with concentration, attention, memory, and judgment. This book presents leading research from around the globe.

Expert Commentary - The hypothesis of a pathway common to the degenerative disease, amenable to particular therapies, is discussed. C3D, formed by activation of the complement cascade, markedly amplifies the synthesis of immunoglobulin, that may increase microglial activation and thus induce neuronal damage and death. If, indeed, the formation of C3D and activated microgliocytes are critical steps in the degenerative pathway, "combination therapy" utilising immunomodulatory and immunosuppressive preparations, the former to inhibit the antigen presenting (dendritic) cell and the latter to inhibit lymphocyte activation, may ameliorate the degenerative process.

Chapter 1 - Multiple sclerosis is a disease of the central nervous system characterised by episodes of neurological dysfunction which often recover, usually followed some years later by progressive and irreversible decline. Lesions of multiple sclerosis are characterised by varying degrees of inflammation, myelin and oligodendrocyte loss, astrogliosis and axonal pathology. Axonal loss is seen in progressive phases of the disease and appears to correlate well with clinical disability. Prior to loss of axons, pathological specimens have revealed changes in the immunohistochemical phenotype of axons. Specifically there may be evidence of dephosphorylation of neurofilaments within axons and transection of axons leading to the formation of axonal spheroids which are rich in dephosphorylated neurofilaments. Evidence of axonal transport defects may also be found in lesions with accumulation of amyloid precursor protein within the axon. Mechanisms of axonal pathology in multiple sclerosis remain unknown, but it is likely that inflammation causes some degree of damage in the acute phases. However, there is evidence that axonal loss may continue even in the absence of inflammation. It has been postulated that axonal loss in this situation occurs due to loss of trophic support from myelin and oligodendrocytes. Oligodendrocytes and myelin are known to provide trophic support for axons and specifically can influence phosphorylated neurofilament levels. The precise mechanisms are unknown, but recent evidence suggests a combination of contact mediated and soluble factors may increase neurofilament phosphorylation and promote axonal protection. Knowledge of such mechanisms may lead to improved therapies to prevent progressive disease. This review will discuss axonal changes in multiple sclerosis, specifically alteration in neurofilament phosphorylation states, and potential mechanisms of axonal protection.

Chapter 2 - Little is known about the proteins involved in axonal damage (AD) which associates with demyelination during multiple sclerosis (MS). Axon transections, amyloid precursor protein accumulation and abnormal expression of the non-phosphorylated form of neurofilaments (NF) have been described. Characterization of AD is a main concern for at least two purposes. First, AD is probably involved in central nervous system (CNS) atrophy, and in patients permanent disability. Second, its impact on remyelination is unknown. Indeed, although neurons are dispensable for oligodendrocytes (OL), the myelinating cells in the CNS, to synthesize myelin-like membranes, neurons enhance this process *in vitro*. Thus, it may be that AD inhibits, in turn, remyelination.

To get insight into these axonal cytoskeleton alterations, the authors have analyzed by immunohistochemistry 18 chronic plaques from autopsy samples, originating from six MS patients (one progressive, five remitting-progressive forms; mean disease duration : 18.5 years). In comparison to the normal appearing white matter, decreased number of axons immunostained for the three NF subunits, βtubulin, and GAP-43 were - with demyelination and loss of oligodendrocytes (OL) - the hallmarks of plaques, and were extremely severe in 2/3. AD intensity did not correlate with demyelination: although severe demyelination always associated with a 90% decrease in NF+ axons, such severe NF loss also occurred in some plaques despite a moderate demyelination, suggesting it depends too upon other factors. and MBP+ OL decreased by the same extent within one plaque, indicating that most OL have reached their final maturation. Nevertheless, residual cells show a lower capability to remyelinate axons, since the ratio of MBP+ fibers per OL decreased also.

These results enlarge previous descriptions of cytoskeleton and NF abnormalities in MS, since the expression of the three subunits of NF are decreased, providing evidence that their intimate constituents are impaired. As previously described in animal models, this decrease could lead to axonal atrophy (and slowness of axon potential conduction). Moreover, severe impairment of NF associates with decreased tubulin expression which could result in altered axoplasmic transport. Finally, one can hypothesize that the expression or localization of NF associated proteins (which copurify with NF) could be altered too.

Thus, the body of these results suggests that NF abnormalities are the core of more severe AD than previously hypothesized in MS. Detailing these lesions will help our understanding of permanent disability in MS patients, as well as cues to prevent them. Whether AD might be involved in MS remyelination impairment – which is one of the actual major target of therapeutic hopes such as cell grafts – is under current investigation at the laboratory.

Chapter 3 - The measurement of functional limitations and disability in individuals with multiple sclerosis (MS) has been plagued by definitional ambiguity and measurement limitations. The abbreviated Late Life-Function and Disability Inventory (LL-FDI) was recently developed based on accepted definitions of functional limitations and disability, and has been preliminarily supported as having good measurement properties in individuals with MS. This study further examined the structural and external aspects of score validity for the LL-FDI in individuals with MS. Individuals with MS completed the LL-FDI and measures of physical activity, walking mobility and neurological impairment. Structural aspects of score validity for the LL-FDI were established using confirmatory factor analysis (CFA). The CFA confirmed the existence of two factors of personal and social aspects of disability for the disability frequency and limitations subscales of the LL-FDI, and three factors of upper extremity function, basic lower extremity function, and advanced lower extremity function for the functional limitations subscale of the LL-FDI. External aspects of score validity for the LL-FDI were established based on expected differences in mean scores between individuals with relapsing-remitting MS and primary and secondary progressive MS and examination of the pattern of correlations between mean scores with the measures of physical activity, walking mobility, and neurological impairment. The authors' results further support the structural and external aspects of score validity for the LL-FDI in individuals with MS, and we recommend that future researchers use this scale when measuring functional limitations and disability in this population.

Chapter 4 - Disease-modifying agents currently used in treatment of multiple sclerosis (MS) are only incompletely effective and are often associated with adverse events and high cost. Thus, alternative treatment options are highly desirable. Statins that are inhibitors of 3-hydroxy-3-methylglutaryl coenzyme A (HMG-CoA) reductase are widely prescribed as cholesterol-lowering agents. They may be a future treatment option for MS – either in an add-on therapy regime or alone – as they have been shown to exhibit potent immunomodulatory effects. Several recent reports have demonstrated that statins prevent and reverse chronic and relapsing experimental autoimmune encephalomyelitis (EAE), an animal model of MS. Furthermore, *in vitro* experiments with human immune cells have exhibited an immunomodulatory mode of action of statins comparable to that of interferon-β. An open label clinical trial assessing simvastatin in MS revealed a significant decrease in the number and volume of new MRI lesions and a favourable safety profile. A large multicenter, placebo-controlled phase II clinical trial assessing atorvastatin in patients with clinically isolated syndrome (CIS; a disease that predisposes to development MS) is currently underway. However, prospective placebo-controlled trials of statins in definite MS are difficult to perform due to ethical and financial objections. Furthermore, overly optimistic reports in the popular media as well as often uncontrolled access of MS patients to statins complicate the evaluation of statins as a realistic treatment option for the future. This chapter reviews the current state of HMG-CoA reductase inhibitors in the context of their putative mechanisms of action and outlines the next steps necessary to increase the level of evidence concerning their therapeutic use in MS.

Chapter 6 – Objectives: On the basis of the authors' and other research on the CD30 molecule, they hypothesized that CD30 may be the unknown molecule involved in the cell contact-dependent suppression of T regulatory cells (Trs) by regulatory dendritic cells (rDCs). Trs are responsible for maintaining the physiological balance between TH1/TH2/TH3 immune responses and central and peripheral tolerance. Thus DC CD30-mediated signals are of key importance both in the initial phase of immune response as well as in maintaining the physiological balance between TH1/TH2/TH3 immune responses. The authors believe that abnormal CD30 signalling can lead to the generation of autoimmune diseases such as multiple sclerosis (MS) and hence, in addition to substantiating the hypothesis above, their objective was also to clarify the immunopathological mechanisms involved in MS and the causes of immunosuppressive drug failure.

Methods: The authors determined network interactions between sCD30, sBcl2 and TH1/TH2/TH3 cytokines (IL12p70, IL12p40, IL10 and TGFβ) in immature (I) DC and DC culture supernatants in IFNβ–1a treated and untreated relapsing-remitting MS (RRMS) patients. TH1/TH2/TH3 cytokine networks in whole blood culture supernatants in PHA activation conditions were also studied.

Results: The overall results, in support of the authors' hypothesis, indicate that CD30 is involved in the cell contact-dependent suppression of TH cells by regulatory IDCs (rIDCs), and rDCs and that this contact-dependent suppression is indispensable for the generation of TGFβ producing Tr (TH3) subsets. Alterations at this level were found in untreated patients, while IFNβ–1a treatment was found to restore the physiological mechanisms by increasing suppressive (sp-) IDC and sp-DC activity (IL10) resulting in a lowering of sCD30 levels, re-establishment of CD30-mediated signals and equilibrium between type1- and type2-like immune response (rICD1/rIDC2 and rDC1/rDC2). Consequently, CD30 being responsible for the balance between Tr1/Tr2, re-establishes equilibrium between immune responses and central and peripheral tolerance. However, it also appears that IFNβ–1a treatment is responsible for the *in vivo* suppression of patient TH1-DC functions which involve the induction of Tr1s for the deletion of self aggressive cells in the immune response in activation conditions, and this may explain the cause of immunosuppressive drug failure.

Conclusion: CD30 mediates signals for a key mechanism involving dendritic and T regulatory cells responsible for maintaining the physiological balance between immune responses and central and peripheral tolerance. Multiple sclerosis is the result of alterations at this level; however, IFNβ-1a treatment is partially successful in restoring the physiological mechanisms affected. Further study can lead to new ways of identifying methods for more effective prevention and treatment of immunopathological conditions such as autoimmune diseases, transplant rejection, allergy and tumor.

Chapter 9 - The changes in emotional and cognitive functioning of patients with MS can be divided into two groups. The first one consists of psychological changes being patients' adaptive reactions to their illness like exogenous depression, neurotic reactions and hypochodrical syndromes. In the second group there are changes caused by the demyelination process (brain damage), for instance, dysfunctions of cognitive and intellectual sphere, and psychiatric syndromes (depression, emotional lability, and uncontrolled crying and laughter). The article focuses on the latter and offers a review of the latest research results on cognitive disorders in multiple sclerosis.

In the beginning the authors present specific cognitive disorders resulting from damages in particular brain locations as well as unspecific cognitive problems caused by the scattered brain damages. Speech impairments, especially dysarrthria, are described most carefully. Moreover, the article provides a report on recent data showing that MS patients suffer also from long and short- term memory impairments and difficulties in learning the new material.

The article contains the characteristics of dementia in the course of MS.

Then the authors discuss the complex relations among four elements: intensity of neurological dysfunctions, clinical course of the multiple sclerosis, its type, and the characteristics of cognitive impairments.

The last part of the article contains a review of the research on the role of neuropsychological tasks and computer programs designed to support the MS patients in their rehabilitiation process aimed to improve their cognitive functioning and prevent, or at least slow down, the further negative changes in this area.

In: Multiple Sclerosis Research Progress
Editors: H. Schwarz, L. Walter
ISBN: 978-1-60456-570-6
© 2008 Nova Science Publishers, Inc.

Expert Commentary

ON THE NATURE OF DEGENERATIVE DISEASES AND POSSIBLE THERAPY: A HYPOTHESIS

Dan G. Milder
Institute of Neurological Sciences, The Prince of Wales Hospital, Sydney, Australia

The hypothesis of a pathway common to the degenerative disease, amenable to particular therapies, is discussed. C3D, formed by activation of the complement cascade, markedly amplifies the synthesis of immunoglobulin, that may increase microglial activation and thus induce neuronal damage and death. If, indeed, the formation of C3D and activated microgliocytes are critical steps in the degenerative pathway, "combination therapy" utilising immunomodulatory and immunosuppressive preparations, the former to inhibit the antigen presenting (dendritic) cell and the latter to inhibit lymphocyte activation, may ameliorate the degenerative process.

INTRODUCTION

Genetic, environmental and immunologic mechanisms are thought to contribute to the degenerative diseases. Purely genetic processes do not explain an usually inexorable progression and predilection for certain sites. Moreover, definite genetic contributions are usually not discernible in the common degenerative diseases. An environmental factor might be expected to result in a "discrete" deficit, that does not progress, or regresses, when the contributory factor is no longer present.

Activated microglia, in areas of neuronal loss, are usually found in the degenerative diseases. Such "activated" microglia are able to elaborate factors, that upregulate the genetic transcription of abnormal proteins and deleterious cytokines, impose oxidative stress and induce apoptosis [1, 2]. Neuronal damage induced by genetic, environmental or immune processes may present to the extracellular environment and hence to immunologic surveillance mechanisms "disrupted" or altered cellular components.

In addition to possible "primary" deleterious effects, such components, either by themselves or by inducing immunoglobulin synthesis, may activate the complement cascade, resulting in the formation of the complement component, C3D. C3D binds covalently to the CD21 (CR2) receptor. By co-ligating the CD21 receptor of B lymphocytes to proteins, C3D greatly amplifies immunoglobulin synthesis by a transduction signal, that activates the CD21/CD19/CD81 cascade [3]. For instance, the attachment of three molecules of C3D to hen egg lysozyme reduces the threshold immunising dose by a factor of 10,000 [4]. Immunoglobulin synthesised by lymphocytes and plasma cells activates microgliocytes by binding to the Fc receptor.

That microglia activated by Fc receptors contribute to disease progression is suggested by the following: immunoglobulin from patients with Parkinson's disease damages dopaminergic cells in culture, [5] and when injected into rat substantia nigra, depletes cells in the pars compacta [6], both effects requiring the microglial Fc gamma receptor; immunoglobulin from patients with motor neuron disease increases calcium and neurotransmitter release from motor neurons in mice, an effect mediated by the microglial Fc gamma receptor [7].

C3D is widely present in the degenerative diseases. It is present, for instance, in the neuritic plaques of Alzheimer's disease, the Lewy bodies of Parkinson's disease, in morphologically intact neurons of motor neuron disease, within the spongiform neuropil of prion disease in "plaque-like" forms, amidst the melanin granules of retinitis pigmentosa, and within the hard and soft exudates of macular degeneration [8-10].

The variable and usually inexorable "progression" of progressive multiple sclerosis mimics that of the degenerations. Disrupted myelin invested by C3D and activated microgliocytes at the edge of long-standing plaques were suggested by Prineas et al. to contribute to disease progression in progressive multiple sclerosis [11]. In an open label study, immunodulatory therapies (one of the three forms in Interferon beta-1b or Glatiramer acetate) and Azathioprine, in combination, were found, in a proportion of patients with progressive forms of multiple sclerosis, to reverse partially visual and neurologic deficits [12, 13]. The effects of such "combination therapy", not present following the administration of either drug alone, might reasonably be the result of actions at separate sites, immunomodulatory therapies possibly inhibiting the antigen presenting (dendritic) cell [14] and Azathioprine lymphocyte activation and hence immunoglobulin synthesis. Quantitative MRI studies in relapsing-remitting multiple sclerosis patients receiving such combination therapy [15] lend support to these observations, that require confirmation by controlled trials.

HYPOTHESIS

If such effects are confirmed and reflected inhibition of C3d synthesis and microglial activation, "combination" therapy may lessen the rate of decline in the degenerative diseases, to which the term "the C3D-microgliocytoses" might be applied. The degree of benefit might vary inversely with the immunogenicity of the antigen. For instance, the intense microgliocytosis of prion disease suggests and immunogenicity increased so greatly as possibly to preclude a therapeutic response. Perhaps, physiologically related systems are antigenically related, a speculation relevant to affection of upper and lower motor neuron elements in motor neuron disease.

"Reversals" in multiple sclerosis, presumably due to a beneficial and possibly regenerative effect upon myelin, would not be expected in the degenerations, in which neurons are unable to regenerate. Progression in disease outside the brain, for instance; glaucoma, in which apoptosis may be a contributory process; cardiomyopathy, in which complement may play a part [16]; and type I diabetes, in which lymphocytic infiltration may not be apparent [17], may also share a similar pathway, possibly amenable to similar therapy.

TESTING THE HYPOTHESIS

Motor neuron disease and Alzheimer's disease are examples in which current methodologies are able to determine, in transgenic animal models and human subjects, in short time spans, a possible therapeutic effect. The possibility of further improvement with the addition of intravenous gamma globulin, able to inhibit the third arm of the pathway, activation of the microglial Fc receptor [18], might also be determined.

ACKNOWLEDGMENTS

A deep sense of gratitude to Professor Sam Berkovic; Professor Peter Blumbergs: Professor Douglas Fearon; Professor Glenda Halliday, Brain Bank, the Prince of Wales Medical Research Institute; Dr. Gregory Hageman, Dr. Renata Kalnins; Dr. Murray Killingworth; Professor John Prineas; Dr. John Sarks; Dr. Shirley Sarks; Professor Jean-Paul Vonsattel, Brain Bank, Columbia-Presbyterian Medical Center; Dr. Tessa Hedley-Whyte, Massachusetts Alzheimer Disease Research Center Brain Bank, Massachusetts General Hospital and Mr. Lawrence Young.

The author has received travel grants from Aventis, Sanofi-Synthelabo, Schering and Serono.

He has no financial interest, direct or otherwise, in the manufacturing or supply of any of the preparations referred to in the text.

REFERENCES

[1] Chen, G., Goeddel, D.V. (2002).TNF-R1 signaling. a beautiful pathway. *Science*, 296,1634-5.

[2] Van Der Laan, L.J., Ruuls, S.R., Weber, K.S. et al. (1996). Macrophage phagocytosis of myelin in vitro determined by flow cytometry: phagocytosis is mediated by Cr3 and induces production of tumour necrosis factor-alpha and nitric oxide. *J Neuroimmunol*, 70,145-52.

[3] Fearon, D.T. (1998).The complement system and adaptive immunity. *Seminars in Immunology*, 10, 355-61.

[4] Dempsey, P.W., Allinson, M.E., Akkaraju, S. et al. (1996).C3d of complement as a molecular adjuvant; bridging innate and acquired immunity. *Science*, 271, 348-50.

[5] Le, W., Rowe, D., Xie, W. et al. (2001).Microglial activation and dopaminergic cell injury: an in vitro model relevant to Parkinson's disease. *J Neurosci*, 21, 8447-55.

[6] He, Y., Le, W.D., Appel, S.H. (2002). Role of Fc gamma receptors in nigral cell injury induced by Parkinson disease immunoglobulin injection into mouse substantia nigra. *Experi Neurol*, 176, 322-7.

[7] Mohamed, H.A., Mosier, D.R., Zou, L.L. et al. (2002).Immunoglobulin Fc gamma receptor promotes immunoglobulin uptake, immunoglobulin-mediated calcium increase, and neurotransmitter release in motor neurons. *J of Neurosci Res*, 69,110-16.

[8] McGeer, P.L., McGeer, E.G., Kawamata, T. et al. (1991).Reactions of the immune system in chronic degenerative neurological diseases. Can J Neurol Sci, 18 (Suppl. 3):376-9.

[9] Yamada, T., McGeer, P.L., McGee, E.G., (1992). Lewy bodies in Parkinson's disease are recognised by antibodies to 9D complement proteins. *Acta Neuropathol*, 84, 100-4.

[10] Hageman, G.S., Luthert, P.J., Victor Chong, N.H. et al. (2001).An integrated hypothesis that considers drusen as biomarkers of immune-mediated processes at the RPE-Bruch's membrane interface in aging and age-related macular degeneration. *Progr Retinal Eye Res*, 20, 705-32.

[11] Prineas, J.W., Kwon, E.E., Cho, E.S. et al. (2001). Immunopathology of secondary-progressive multiple sclerosis. *Ann Neurol*, 50, 646-57.

[12] Milder, D.G. (2002). Partial and significant reversal of progressive visual and neurologic deficits in multiple sclerosis: a possible ther- apeutic effect. *Clini Experi Ophthalmol*, 30, 363-6.

[13] Milder, D.G. (2002).Immunomodulatory therapies and low dose Azathioprine reverse partially and significantly progressive visual and neurologic deficits in multiple sclerosis: further observations. *Acta Myol*, 21,144-50.

[14] Hussien, Y., Sanna, A., Soderdstrom, M. et al. (2001). Glatiramer acetate and IFN-beta act on dendritic cells in multiple sclerosis. *J of Neuroimmunol*, 121,102-10.

[15] Markovic-Plese, S., Bielekova, B., Kadom, N. et al. (2003).Longitu dinal magnetic resonance imaging study on the effect of Azathioprine in relapsing-remitting multiple sclerosis refractory to the treatment with Interferon B-1b. *Neurology*, 60,1849-51.

[16] Kaya Z, Afanasyeva M, Wang Y, et al. (2001).Contribution of the innate immune system to autoimmune myocarditis: a role for complement. *Nature Immunol*, 2, 739-45.

[17] Hanafusa T, Miyazaki A, Miyagawa J, et al. (1990). Examination of islets in the pancreas biopsy specimens from newly diag nosed type 1 (insulin-dependent) diabetic patients. *Diabetologia*, 33,105-11.

[18] Basta M, Dalakas, M.C. (1994). High-dose Intravenous immunoglobulin exerts its beneficial effect in patients with dermatomyositis by blocking endomysial deposition of activated complement fragments. *J Clin Invest*, 94, 1729-35.

In: Multiple Sclerosis Research Progress
Editors: H. Schwarz, L. Walter

ISBN: 978-1-60456-570-6
© 2008 Nova Science Publishers, Inc.

Chapter 1

NEUROFILAMENT CHANGES IN MULTIPLE SCLEROSIS

Alastair Wilkins**[*]**
Department of Clinical Neurosciences and Centre for Brain Repair,
University of Cambridge, Forvie Site, Robinson Way, Cambridge, UK

ABSTRACT

Multiple sclerosis is a disease of the central nervous system characterised by episodes of neurological dysfunction which often recover, usually followed some years later by progressive and irreversible decline. Lesions of multiple sclerosis are characterised by varying degrees of inflammation, myelin and oligodendrocyte loss, astrogliosis and axonal pathology. Axonal loss is seen in progressive phases of the disease and appears to correlate well with clinical disability. Prior to loss of axons, pathological specimens have revealed changes in the immunohistochemical phenotype of axons. Specifically there may be evidence of dephosphorylation of neurofilaments within axons and transection of axons leading to the formation of axonal spheroids which are rich in dephosphorylated neurofilaments. Evidence of axonal transport defects may also be found in lesions with accumulation of amyloid precursor protein within the axon. Mechanisms of axonal pathology in multiple sclerosis remain unknown, but it is likely that inflammation causes some degree of damage in the acute phases. However, there is evidence that axonal loss may continue even in the absence of inflammation. It has been postulated that axonal loss in this situation occurs due to loss of trophic support from myelin and oligodendrocytes. Oligodendrocytes and myelin are known to provide trophic support for axons and specifically can influence phosphorylated neurofilament levels. The precise mechanisms are unknown, but recent evidence suggests a combination of contact mediated and soluble factors may increase neurofilament phosphorylation and promote axonal protection. Knowledge of such mechanisms may lead to improved

[*] Correspondence: Alastair Wilkins, Department of Clinical Neurosciences and Centre for Brain Repair, University of Cambridge, Forvie Site, Robinson Way, Cambridge CB2 2PY UK Tel: +44 1223 331186, Fax: +44 1223 331174; e-mail: aw255@cam.ac.uk

therapies to prevent progressive disease. This review will discuss axonal changes in multiple sclerosis, specifically alteration in neurofilament phosphorylation states, and potential mechanisms of axonal protection.

ABBREVIATIONS

BDNF	brain-derived neurotrophic factor
CNPase	2',3'-cyclic nucleotide 3'-phosphodiesterase
CNS	central nervous system
CSF	cerebrospinal fluid
GDNF	glial cell-line derived neurotrophic factor
IF	intermediate filament
IGF-1	insulin-like growth factor type-1
MAG	myelin associated glycoprotein
MBP	myelin basic protein
MOG	myelin-oligodendrocyte glycoprotein
NF	neurofilament
NGF	nerve growth factor
NO	nitric oxide
PLP	proteolipid protein

INTRODUCTION

Multiple sclerosis is a common disease of the central nervous system (CNS) which presents significant challenges to the clinician treating the disease and scientists researching it. Once thought the archetypal inflammatory CNS disorder, evidence now suggests the pathophysiology is complex and possibly occurs via multiple mechanisms including neurodegeneration (Compston, 2006). The complexity of the disease is born out by the inadequacy of current treatments; and the progressive phase of the disease, during which patients accrue disability relentlessly, has no effective therapy.

Axon pathology in multiple sclerosis was first described by Charcot in his classical reports of the disease over 100 years ago, but the focus on inflammatory demyelinating plaques and their pathogenesis led to a paucity of research on the subject until several reports in the late 1990s re-emphasised this aspect of pathology. Most notably, Trapp and colleagues (1998) demonstrated axonal transection and changes in neurofilament phosphorylation states in axons within acute lesions of multiple sclerosis. Subsequent work has shown further axonal changes and has revealed that axonal loss belies progression of the disease.

This review will discuss the evidence behind axonal pathology in multiple sclerosis, focusing on neurofilament changes; discuss potential mechanisms of the process and possible neuroprotective therapies in the disease.

The Natural History of Multiple Sclerosis

Multiple sclerosis is generally characterised by episodes of acute neurological dysfunction which usually recover, followed at some stage by slow and insidious progression and development of fixed neurological deficits (Compston and Coles, 2002). Most patients experience an initial relapsing and remitting preliminary course of the disease. During such relapses neurological dysfunction is thought to be due to the effect of inflammatory cytokines and conduction block resulting from disruption of myelin (Coles et al., 1999). Myelin is produced by oligodendrocytes in the central nervous system and allows for rapid saltatory conduction to occur via the formation of nodes of Ranvier. At such nodes there is grouping of sodium channels allowing for efficient action potential propagation. Furthermore myelin itself offers high resistance and low capacitance which again improves saltatory conduction. In the absence of myelin, axonal conduction is severely impaired and conduction of electrical impulses between internodes fails by virtue of myelin loss and a redistribution of sodium channels along the length of the axon (Craner et al., 2003; Craner et al., 2004).

Mechanisms for remission from attacks are rather poorly understood, but involve resolution of inflammation, reorganisation of axonal channels and limited remyelination (Smith et al., 1979). Indeed current therapies for the disease aim at reducing inflammation during the acute phase of the disease with drugs such as β-interferon (Jacobs et al., 2000). However most patients, in due course, will enter a phase of the disease in which remission does not occur and the disease progresses inexorably. During this progressive phase of the disease disability correlates with radiological markers of axon loss, including magnetic resonance spectroscopic analysis of NAA and brain atrophy (Davie et al., 1997). Reasons as to why remission does not occur at this stage of the disease are the subject of extensive research, but a long-term failure of remyelination and lack of a supportive environment for the axon seem likely. Failure of effective remyelination is thought to be due to depletion of remyelinating cells, quiescence of oligodendrocyte precursor cells and axonal inhibitory signals (Lubetzki et al., 2005).

At the present time once the progressive phase of the disease has been entered, there are no effective therapies for the disease, which would appear to reflect the inability of therapeutic agents to prevent axonal degeneration. Indeed a striking failure of current treatments for multiple sclerosis has been there poor efficacy in preventing accumulation of disability in later stages of the disease (Kappos, 2004). The main reason for this appears to relate to the mode of action of drugs such as β-interferon which target the inflammatory response. Epidemiological data concerning multiple sclerosis has, however, shown that inflammation is unlikely to be the sole cause for clinical deterioration in the progressive phases of the disease.

Specifically the European database for multiple sclerosis (EDMUS) database has been highly informative. This has revealed that once a certain level of disability has been reached in patient cohorts, further disease progression occurs at the same rate in those who do not have superimposed relapses, compared to those who do (Confavreux et al., 2000). This is in contrast to the clinical course early in the disease process, which does seem to be dependent on relapse rate in determining early disease rate. More recent evidence has suggested that there may be dissociation of the inflammatory and degenerative processes even from disease onset, as evidenced by similarities in rates of progression of those patients with primary progressive disease, in which the disease does not commence with a period of relapses and remissions, and those with secondary progressive disease (Confavreux and Vukusic, 2006). Furthermore evidence from treatment trials concurs with the concept that disease progression may be partially independent of inflammatory activity. CAMPATH-1H, a humanised monoclonal antibody, is highly effective in abolishing inflammatory relapses in patients with multiple sclerosis, but has no effect on disease progression in those patients with existing disability (Coles et al., 1999).

From these studies has emerged, therefore, the notion of two processes occurring during the pathogenesis of multiple sclerosis. The idea that the inflammatory and the neurodegenerative processes may run in parallel and may be independent of each other challenges existing concepts about the disease and the way in which it should be treated. The search for therapies which tackle the neurodegenerative component of disease progression is an important concept. At the heart of this is the need to understand axonal pathology in the disease and mechanisms underlying axon protection.

Axonal Pathology in MS

The classic histological features of acute lesions of multiple sclerosis include perivascular infiltrates of small lymphocytes, loss of myelin and oligodendrocytes, myelin-laden macrophages and axonal damage (Frohman et al., 2006). However there may be extensive variability between lesions. Some authors have recognised 4 distinct types of acute lesions based on pathological studies (Lucchinetti et al., 1996; Lucchinetti et al., 2000). These types are felt to reflect potential heterogeneity in disease pathogenesis. Patterns I and II show similarities to T-cell-mediated or T-cell plus antibody-mediated autoimmune encephalomyelitis. Type I is characterised by demyelination and the presence of macrophages and cytokines, such as tumour necrosis factor-α (TNFα). Type II is similar but shows immunoglobulin and complement activity. Type III, in contrast, lacks immunoglobulin deposition, but shows oligodendrocyte dysfunction and demyelination, whereas type IV is characterised by oligodendrocyte apoptosis through DNA fragmentation. Thus types III and IV are suggestive of a primary oligodendrocyte dystrophy, reminiscent of virus- or toxin-induced demyelination rather than autoimmunity. The reasons for these differences and the importance in disease phenotypes have yet to be determined. However, a further demyelinating disease of the central nervous system, Devic's disease or neuromyelitis optica, which is a distinct variant from multiple sclerosis shows marked antibody mediated tissue injury, is characterised by the presence of a specific circulating antibody in the serum and typically responds to plasma exchange therapy (Scolding, 2005). This pathological and phenotypic subtype of CNS demyelination with a good response to a certain therapy distinguishes it from other inflammatory disease and raises the future possibility of tailoring therapies to immunopathological subtypes of disease.

In chronic active lesions of MS the histological appearances may be somewhat different with hypertophic astocytes and degenerating axons, as well as perivascular cuffs of infiltrating cells and lipid-laden macrophages. These lesions may show some degree of remyelination and recruitment of cells of the oligodendrocyte lineage, although remyelination is generally poor and incomplete (Dubois-Dalq et al. 2005). This failure of repair in chronic lesions is thought to be a major reason for disease progression and much active research is targeted at attempts to enhance remyelination (Zhao et al., 2005). Chronic inactive lesions of MS are characterised by astrogliosis, a paucity of oligodendrocytes and reduced numbers of demyelinated axons.

Axonal pathology was described by Charcot in his initial histopathological descriptions of the disease at the end of the nineteenth century, but it was not until over one hundred years later that the subject of axonopathy in MS became the focus of active research. Histopathological analyses of chronic multiple sclerosis lesions have revealed significant reductions in axon density (Lovas et al., 2000; DeLuca et al., 2004). In addition, a number of axonal markers have now been used which highlight dysfunction of the axon prior to degeneration. The two markers in commonest use are: amyloid precursor protein accumulation (APP) and the presence of dephosphorylated neurofilaments.

APP is rapidly transported down axons and normal axons do not stain for the protein. The presence of APP staining in axon tracts implies disruption of fast axonal transport and thus dysfunction of the axon. APP accumulation occurs in both acute active lesions and in chronic lesions of MS (Ferguson et al., 1997; Bitsch et al., 2000; Kuhlmann et al., 2002). APP accumulation may also occur in 'normal appearing white matter' of multiple sclerosis tissue, which has again added to evidence that axonopathy maybe widespread and not exclusively related to inflammation (Kornek et al., 2000). However, APP accumulation within axons is most marked within active inflammatory lesions and appears to correlate with numbers of infiltrating inflammatory cells (Bitsch et al., 2000). It may be, therefore, that APP accumulation within axons is marking acute disruption of axonal function and may be the earliest sign of axonal dysfunction within a lesion. It is unknown the extent to which the process of APP accumulation within axons is reversible, but this concept is likely to be of vital importance when considering potential therapies for axonopathy in the disease.

Neurofilament dephosphorylation within axons has been well documented in multiple sclerosis and will be discussed in detail below.

Other axonal changes have been reported, notably changes in ion channel distribution. In normal myelinated axons sodium channels are clustered at high density at nodes of Ranvier, facilitating effective saltatory conduction. Recent work on sodium channel distribution in MS tissue has revealed changes in channel distributions associated with areas of axonal injury (Craner *et al.,* 2004). In axons positive for APP staining, corresponding to axonal dysfunction, the sodium channel subtype ($Na_v1.6$) which usually clusters at the node of Ranvier is found rather diffusely along the axon. Furthermore the channel co-localises with the sodium/calcium exchanger. Increased and persistent sodium influx through $Na_v1.6$ channels may then lead to reversal of the sodium/channel exchange mechanism and an accumulation of intraxonal calcium, leading to axonal injury (Waxman et al., 2004). Indeed similar mechanisms have been postulated in experimental models of inflammatory central nervous system disease. Rat dorsal roots exposed to nitric oxide degenerate when electrically activated, a process which is attenuated by sodium channel blockers, such as flecainide (Smith et al., 2000; Kapoor et al., 2003).

Axonal dysfunction can also be studied by other techniques. Great advances have been made in recent years in imaging the brain and spinal cord. This has led to greater diagnostic clarity but has also provided insight into pathophysiological processes that may be occurring throughout the duration of the disease. Specifically, magnetic resonance spectroscopy (MRS) is a technique which allows quantification of certain tissue metabolites in the brains of live patients. N-acetyl aspartate (NAA) is found predominantly in neurons and the spectroscopic detection of the compound is a marker of axonal density in the nervous system (Bjartmar et al., 2000). Reductions in brain NAA levels have been detected in acute active lesions of MS, chronic active lesions and so-called normal appearing white matter (NAWM) of patients with the disease (Davie et al., 1995; Leary et al., 1999). Furthermore persistent neurological disability correlates to reductions in NAA levels, an observation which has led to the hypothesis that permanent disability in MS is caused by axonal loss. An '*in vivo*' marker of axonal integrity is a vital component of future trials which aim to address neurodegenerative processes in the disease.

Indeed, the search for 'biomarkers' in multiple sclerosis has been intense in an attempt to correlate potential therapies with effects on pathology in patients. One such marker is the presence of neurofilaments with the cerebrospinal fluid (CSF; Petzold, 2005). It has been postulated that the presence of these molecules within the CSF may be an indicator of axon destruction within the CNS: when axons degenerate neurofilaments are released into the extracellular fluid space and from there enter the CSF. The precise relationship between CSF concentrations of neurofilaments and the degree of axonal degeneration is unknown. Although more work is required on changes in neurofilament levels in the CSF as the disease progresses, there is a suggestion that levels increase during progressive phases of multiple sclerosis (Petzold et al., 2005).

NEUROFILAMENTS AND MS

As discussed, changes in neurofilament phosphorylation states have been detected in axons and taken as evidence of pathological dysfunction. Below I will discuss axonal structure, changes in neurofilament phosphorylation levels in multiple sclerosis and the influence of myelin and oligodendrocytes on neurofilament phosphorylation in relation to putative changes occurring in multiple sclerosis.

The axonal cytoskeleton is composed of scaffolding filaments: actin microfilaments, microtubules and intermediate filaments (IFs). Neurofilaments (NFs) are neuron-specific IFs which consist of three subunits – a light chain (NF-L), a medium chain (NF-M) and a heavy chain (NF-H) differing in molecular weight by virtue of their hypervariable tail domains (Fuchs and Weber, 1994). The C-terminal region of NF-M and NF-H contain 10-15 and 40-50 lysine-serine-proline (KSP) repeats respectively acting as potential phosphorylation sites (Veeranna *et al.,* 1998). NF-H is the most extensively phosphorylated protein in the human brain and the process of phosphorylation and dephosphorylation is highly complex. In brief, phosphorylation occurs via a number of kinases and is predominantly regulated within the axonal compartment (Grant and Pant, 2000). During development, NF phosphorylation appears to be a key factor in triggering NF accumulation and thus the formation of axons (Sanchez et al., 2000). Phosphorylation of NFs also leads to slowing of NF transport, promotion of NF alignment and an increase in inter-NF spacing, all of which contribute to axon structure, function and stability (Leterrier et al., 1996; Yabe et al., 2001). Virtually all NF-H KSP sites in mature, healthy axons are phosphorylated *in vivo*, a process which occurs exclusively in axons (Elhanany et al., 1994).

Neurofilaments are slowly transported down the axon and the velocity of transport is inversely proportional to degree of phosphorylation (Nixon et al., 1994). It is thought that when neurofilaments reach the axon terminus they are then degraded through protease dependent mechanisms. High levels of phosphorylation within neurofilaments are however protective against proteolysis (Goldstein et al., 1987). The corollary to which suggests that neurofilaments that have become dephosphorylated may be more susceptible to proteolytic damage and thus degeneration of the axon. Whether this process underlies axon degeneration in multiple sclerosis is unknown.

Neurofilament dephosphorylation has been used as a marker for axonal pathology in multiple sclerosis and in experimental models of demyelination. The precise relationship between neurofilament dephosphorylation and axonal degeneration is not known. Nor is it known exactly why neurofilaments become dephosphorylated.

Antibodies directed against different phosphoisoforms of neurofilament have been used to study the process in multiple sclerosis. Most commonly, antibodies against dephosphorylated neurofilaments (SMI32; Sternberger Monoclonals, USA) have been used and shown to mark axonal abnormalities in the disease (Trapp et al., 1998). In this study, neurofilament dephosphorylation was seen in both active inflammatory lesions and also in chronic active lesions. SMI32 also marked terminal axonal swelling or 'spheroids' which represent transected axons and thus irreversible axonal destruction. Interestingly, quantification of terminal axonal spheroids identified a strong correlation between axonal transection and the inflammatory activity of the lesion. This provides evidence that axonopathy in the disease may occur early and be related, to some extent, to inflammation.

Mechanisms of inflammatory axon destruction are likely to be complex, but a role for nitric oxide (NO) has emerged from experimental studies. NO serves many physiological functions within the nervous system, including roles in synaptic plasticity, long-term potentiation and neurotransmitter release, but at sites of inflammation high concentrations of NO are thought to mediate cell death (Smith and Lassmann, 2002). Microglial derived NO has been shown to be neurotoxic *in vitro* (Bal-Price and Brown, 2001; Golde et al., 2001). Mechanisms underlying this neurotoxicity are complex, but NO activates a number of intracellular signaling pathways including MAPkinases and may ultimately lead to neuronal death via inhibition of mitochondrial respiration (Brown and Borutaite, 2002; Ghatan et al., 2000). Recent *in vivo* work has shown that NO may also mediate activity dependent axon destruction (Smith et al., 2001). Furthermore pathological studies have demonstrated activity of inducible nitric oxide sythetase (iNOS) within acute inflammatory lesions of multiple sclerosis (Bagasra et al., 1995).

NO has also been shown to have effects on neurofilament phosphorylation levels within axons in culture (Wilkins and Compston, 2005). In this system, activation of p38 MAPkinase by NO leads to axonal destruction and reduced levels of phosphorylated neurofilaments (via inhibition of MAPkinase/Erk signaling). Activation of MAPkinase/Erk and inhibition of p38 MAPkinase signaling by growth factors lead to attenuation of NO mediated axonal destruction.

Evidence for chronic axonal attrition has accumulated in recent years with pathological studies demonstrating reduction in axonal densities in chronic inactive plaques (Lovas et al., 2000; DeLuca et al., 2004). It is unclear whether axon drop-out occurs in these late stages as a result of previous inflammatory damage to axons; as a result of low grade inflammation occurring causing damage to already vulnerable demyelinated axons; as a result of loss of trophic environment for axons to survive; or as part of a completely independent neurodegenerative process. Indeed recent evidence has shown that there may be poor correlation between plaque load and axon loss in post-mortem specimens of multiple sclerosis tissue (deLuca et al., 2006). Certain axonal tracts also appear more susceptible to injury in multiple sclerosis (deLuca et al., 2004). These studies, although only providing a 'snap shot' of a dynamic disease, argue that demyelination is not the primary determinant of axon loss and axonal degeneration may be driven by non-inflammatory mechanisms.

How to tie up these seemingly disparate pathological mechanisms? One might hypothesise that inflammation, causing widespread tissue damage, contributes to early axon destruction via molecules such as nitric oxide. However, destruction of oligodendrocytes and myelin also occurs at this stage and may 'set up' the later process of chronic axonal drop-out. Myelin mutant studies have shown that myelin is an important determinant of long term axonal survival (see below). Thus myelin and oligodendrocyte loss may leave axons particularly susceptible to degeneration via this mechanism. Furthermore such axons may be rendered particularly susceptible to very low levels of inflammation. This may account for the lack of correlation between inflammation and axon loss in later stages of the disease. Thus the microenvironment of the axon may be critical to determine its capacity for long term survival. In other words, there may be a balance between the deleterious effects of inflammation and other toxic mediators and the trophic axonoprotective environment of surrounding cells. Once that balance is tipped towards favouring toxic inflammation, axon degeneration may proceed inexorably. The goals of axonoprotective treatments, therefore, may be to tip the balance in the opposite direction by restoring the trophic environment surrounding the axon.

Oligodendrocyte Influences on Axonal Survival and Neurofilament Phosphorylation

Thus, one interpretation for post-inflammatory axon loss is that the environment in which axons find themselves is no longer sufficient supportive to maintain them. Specifically the severe loss of myelin and oligodendrocytes within chronic lesions may lead to an environment in which the axon lacks necessary survival factors. Indeed there has been increasing evidence for an axonotrophic role of central nervous system myelin. Furthermore oligodendrocytes have been shown to produce soluble growth factors which influence the survival and phenotype of axons. The evidence for these phenomena will be discussed.

Myelin Has Neurotrophic Properties

Myelin has neurotrophic properties in both the peripheral and central nervous system, although mechanisms differ in these two sites (Yin et al., 2006). Myelin mutants have provided insights into processes by which myelin is important in axon development and maintenance. However, caution should be exercised when translating the study of myelin mutants to consider chronic progressive stages of multiple sclerosis as axons of mutant animals are exposed to abnormal myelin throughout their life.

In the peripheral nervous system, Schwann cells influence peripheral axonal structure, as hypomyelinating sciatic nerves show marked reductions in NF phosphorylation and density, with associated decrease in axonal calibre (Cole et al., 1994). These nerves show no changes in total NF content, suggesting Schwann cell myelin has direct influences on the process of neurofilament phosphorylation. In a similar way, mice deficient in myelin-associated glycoprotein (MAG) have reduced peripheral axonal calibres, reduced NF phosphorylation and decreased inter-NF spacing, again implying a role for myelin components in NF regulation within the peripheral nervous system (Yin et al., 1998).

In the central nervous system, myelin also significantly influences axon development. Central myelin is composed of several proteins including proteolipid protein (PLP) and DM20 (an alternate spliced isoform), myelin basic protein (MBP), myelin associated glycoprotein (MAG), myelin-oligodendrocyte glycoprotein (MOG) and 2',3'-cyclic nucleotide 3'-phosphodiesterase (CNPase). The absence of central myelin leads to severe disability and pronounced axonal dystrophy, as demonstrated by the *Shiverer* mouse which contains a deletion in the MBP gene and thus produces no MBP protein. This leads to the complete absence of compact CNS myelin and a phenotype of tremor and seizures with decreased life span of the mice. CNS axonal changes occur within these animals, including an increase in slow axonal transport, microtubule density and number, and altered neurofilament assembly and phosphorylation (Brady et al., 1999; Sanchez et al., 2000; Kirkpatrick et al., 2001). The effect appears dose dependent, since mice expressing 25% of wild-type MBP, with thin compact myelin sheaths, show an intermediate phenotype.

Mice containing other mutations in myelin proteins have been produced which show abnormalities in structure of the myelin, but nevertheless some degree of myelination. These mutants may help understand which particular components of myelin are important in the long term maintenance of axons.

PLP is localised predominantly in compact myelin and is its major structural component. Interestingly, mice lacking the Plp gene (X chromosome) are able to synthesise large amounts of myelin, which only show morphological defects in the interperiod line (the area in compact myelin where external leaflets of two adjacent plasma membranes are closely apposed). These mice do however show impairment of axonal transport mechanisms and late onset axonal degeneration with 'ovoid' formation (Griffiths et al., 1998b; Edgar et al., 2004). Interestingly, it appears that axons may become dependent on oligodendrocyte support sometime after myelination has been completed, as non-myelinated axons within optic nerves from chimeric females (which show patches of normally myelinated and non-myelinated axons) never develop axonal swellings over the expected time course. This implies a role for PLP in maintaining axons that have become oligodendrocyte dependent, although the signal triggering this putative dependency remains unknown. Further studies of chimeric females have revealed a role for PLP in early stages of axon-oligodendrocyte interactions, initiating the ensheathment and myelination of a proportion of small-diameter axons (Yool et al., 2001). The specific role for PLP in the central nervous system has been highlighted by a recent report in which mice were engineered to express the peripheral myelin component P_0 instead of PLP centrally (Yin et al., 2006). Mice lacking PLP (but expressing P_0 centrally) show a structure and periodicity of myelin which resembled peripheral myelin, yet had severe disability and degeneration of myelinated axons. Those mice expressing equal amounts of PLP and P_0 show normal phenotype and no axonal degeneration. This implies a specific role of central nervous system myelin (containing PLP) in neuroprotection of central axons, and highlights the differences between the requirements of central and peripheral axons.

Another example of the differences between central and peripheral axonal requirements comes from the study of mice lacking MAG. Axonal abnormalities are not a prominent feature within the central nervous system of these mice, whereas chronic atrophy, changes in calibre and alterations in neurofilament organization of peripheral axons occur (Li et al., 1994; Yin et al., 1998).

CNPase, a further structural molecule of myelin, has also been shown to have a role in axon-glial interactions (Lappe-Siefke et al., 2003). Mice lacking CNPase have morphologically normal myelin, but show delayed axonal swelling and degeneration, again suggesting that specific interactions between myelin components and the axon may determine long-term survival of the axon.

These studies suggest that the presence of structurally normal myelin may be required for long term axonal survival and that its absence will lead to chronic and slow axonal dropout. Whether this translates to the pathophysiology of axonal degeneration in chronic demyelinated lesions is unclear. Axons within myelin mutants are never exposed to structurally normal myelin, and so may develop different trophic requirements to axons ensheathed with structurally normal myelin.

As outlined, influences of myelin on neurofilament phosphorylation have been shown although the exact influence of individual myelin protein on the process are unclear. Furthermore the mechanism by which neurofilaments become dephosphorylated following demyelination is unknown.

Oligodendrocyte Derived Growth Factors Influence Axonal Survival and Neurofilament Phosphorylation

Growth factors have effects on neurofilament phosphorylation levels and there is increasing evidence that growth factors released by oligodendrocytes may influence axonal phenotype in this way. The close proximity of the oligodendrocyte to the axon would imply the possibility of cross talk between the two cell types. Indeed axon-derived factors are known to influence oligodendrocytes in a way which leads to effective functioning of glial-neuronal sub-units.

Neurons secrete factors which influence oligodendrocyte behaviour and phenotype. Specifically axons have been shown to exert a proliferative effect on oligodendrocyte precursor cells. This was first shown by transection studies on the rat neonatal optic nerve (David et al., 1984). Experimental transection of axons leads to a decrease in the yield of oligodendrocytes that may be cultured from the nerve. Several factors have subsequently been identified as being important in this process, including PDGF, basic FGF and members of the neuregulin family (Bogler et al., 1990; Canoll et al., 1996). Axons also promote oligodendrocyte survival (Barres and Raff, 1999). This observation is inferred from several studies of post-natal optic nerve transection . For instance, cutting the P8 optic nerve behind the eye leads to a fourfold increase in oligodendrocyte apoptosis, detected three days after transection (Barres et al., 1993). However, oligodendrocyte death induced by transection of the optic nerve is abrogated by locally elevated neuregulin concentrations (Fernandez et al., 2000). Neuregulins (Ngr1) are also crucially important in determining myelin sheath thickness and matching it to axon diameter (Michailov et al., 2004). Thus, signaling between neurons and cells of the oligodendrocyte lineage appears to be important in matching oligodendrocyte numbers to axonal surface area and also in ensuring that the correct cellular substrates are in place before the onset of myelination and formation of mature myelinating units.

In a similar way oligodendrocytes secrete soluble factors which influence axonal survival and phenotype. This phenomenon has been elucidated by a series of *in vitro* experiments, and there significance *in vivo* has yet to be fully identified (Du and Dreyfus, 2002). Compared to well documented and extensive studies of astrocyte-derived neurotrophic production, oligodendrocytes have traditionally been considered to be less important providers of such factors in the central nervous system.

Byravan et al., (1994) initially showed nerve growth factor (NGF) and brain-derived neurotrophic factor (BDNF) mRNA production by an immortalized oligodendrocyte cell line. This observation was prompted by observations of the ability of this line to promote neurite extension in PC12 cells. Furthermore, these workers showed co-localisation of NGF protein in both oligodendrocyte precursor cells and mature oligodendrocytes. A later study showed expression of NGF, BDNF and neurotrophin-3 (NT-3) mRNA in cultures of basal forebrain oligodendrocytes (Dai et al., 2003). Expression of these mRNAs may be altered by factors such as glutamate and potassium, suggesting that neuronal signals may provide feedback to regulate oligodendrocyte-mediated neurotrophism. Furthermore, Shinar and McMorris (1995) showed insulin-like growth factor type-1 (IGF-1) mRNA production by cultured oligodendrocytes. An extensive study of glial cell-line derived neurotrophic factor (GDNF) family member mRNA production in cells of oligodendrocyte lineage has shown GDNF mRNA production in oligodendrocyte cell line and within differentiated primary oligodendrocyte cultures (Strelau and Unsicker, 1999).

The functional significance of these findings has been shown by several studies suggesting that oligodendrocyte derived factors improve the survival of neurons and, more specifically, axons in culture. Meyer-Franke et al., (1995) detected an as yet uncharacterised soluble protein of >30kDa derived from mature oligodendrocytes that improved the survival of post-natal retinal ganglion cells. Later studies confirmed IGF-1 production by cells of the oligodendrocyte lineage and oligodendrocyte derived IGF-1 improves the survival of stressed neurons under conditions of trophic factor deprivation (Wilkins et al., 2001). Furthermore oligodendrocyte derived factors also increase levels of phosphorylated neurofilament within cultured neurons and thus aid axonal survival under the same conditions of trophic factor deprivation (Wilkins et al., 2003). Specifically, GDNF is the growth factor that appears to be of importance in this phenomenon and GDNF is only produced by differentiated oligodendrocytes and not precursor cells. GDNF promotes increased levels of neurofilament phosphorylation via MAPkinase/ Erk signalling pathways, as inhibition of this pathway attenuates the process and GDNF strongly activates Erk signalling within neurons. Mechanisms by which neurofilaments become phosphorylated are complex, but a role for MAPkinase /Erk has been established (Pang et al., 1995; Veerana et al., 1998; Li et al., 1999). Using a similar approach, oligodendrocyte derived growth factors and GDNF has also been shown to attenuate nitric oxide mediated destruction of axons, again via MAPkinase /Erk signaling (Wilkins and Compston, 2005). Again, addition of these factors significantly increases levels of phosphorylated neurofilament within cultured axons. Furthermore this study emphasises the interaction of several different signalling pathways which are involved in neuroprotective activities. p38 MAPkinase is strongly activated by addition of nitric oxide to neurons, yet inhibiton of p38 leads to activation of MAPkinase /Erk pathways. This implies a central role for Erk activation in protection of axons from inflammatory insults.

These studies have shown considerable neurotrophic and axonotrophic effects of oligodendrocytes. Both myelin and oligodendrocyte derived growth factors exert influences on long-term neuronal survival, specifically of the axonal subunit, and influence neurofilament phosphorylation within the axon.

Conclusion

Axon loss and dysfunction underlies clinical progression in multiple sclerosis. Understanding of the mechanisms involved in the process of axonopathy is vital in order to devise therapies which address specific pathophysiological processes. The concept of several mechanisms occurring within the time course of the disease probably belies the failure of current therapies which only address the inflammatory phase of the disease. Non-inflammatory processes are likely to be important in later stages of the disease and may be responsible clinical disease progression to a large degree. This 'neurodegenerative' phase of the disease is now a major target for research and in the coming years treatments will need to address this aspect. Potential treatments include remyelination therapies, delivery of growth factors or neuroprotectant drug therapies. Of these, remyelination has been the subject of extensive research. In theory, remyelination has the potential to address many aspects of disease pathology and offers the hope of recovery from symptoms. In reality, the choice of remyelinating cell, achieving satisfactory remyelination and targeting multiple lesions which are widely disseminated in space, are major obstacles preventing it becoming an imminent therapeutic option. Drugs and growth factor treatments which address axon degeneration and neurofilament dephosphorylation also seem likely to become attractive additions to the clinician's range of options available to treat patients with progressive disease. With the expansion in knowledge concerning axon pathology in multiple sclerosis such treatment options may not be far away.

References

Bagasra O, Michaels FH, Zheng YM et al., Activation of the inducible form of nitric oxide synthase in the brains of patients with multiple sclerosis. *Proc.Natl.Acad.Sci.U.S.A* 1995; 92: 12041-12045.

Bal-Price A, Brown GC. Inflammatory neurodegeneration mediated by nitric oxide from activated glia-inhibiting neuronal respiration, causing glutamate release and excitotoxicity. *J.Neurosci. 2001;* 21: 6480-6491.

Barres BA, Jacobson MD, Schmid R, Sendtner M, Raff MC. Does oligodendrocyte survival depend on axons? *Curr.Biol. 1993;* 3: 489-497.

Barres BA, Raff MC. Axonal control of oligodendrocyte development. *J.Cell Biol. 1999;* 147: 1123-1128.

Bitsch A, Schuchardt J, Bunkowski S, Kuhlmann T, Bruck W. Acute axonal injury in multiple sclerosis. Correlation with demyelination and inflammation. *Brain 2000;* 123 (Pt 6): 1174-1183.

Bjartmar C, Kidd G, Mork S, Rudick R, Trapp BD. Neurological disability correlates with spinal cord axonal loss and reduced N-acetyl aspartate in chronic multiple sclerosis patients. *Ann.Neurol. 2000;* 48: 893-901.

Bogler O, Wren D, Barnett SC, Land H, Noble M. Cooperation between two growth factors promotes extended self-renewal and inhibits differentiation of oligodendrocyte-type-2 astrocyte (O-2A) progenitor cells. *Proc.Natl.Acad.Sci.U.S.A 1990;* 87: 6368-6372.

Brady ST, Witt AS, Kirkpatrick LL et al., Formation of compact myelin is required for maturation of the axonal cytoskeleton. *J.Neurosci. 1999;* 19: 7278-7288.

Brown GC, Borutaite V. Nitric oxide inhibition of mitochondrial respiration and its role in cell death. *Free Radic.Biol.Med. 2002;* 33: 1440-1450.

Byravan S, Foster LM, Phan T, Verity AN, Campagnoni AT. Murine oligodendroglial cells express nerve growth factor. *Proc.Natl.Acad.Sci.U.S.A 1994;* 91: 8812-8816.

Canoll PD, Musacchio JM, Hardy R, Reynolds R, Marchionni MA, Salzer JL. GGF/neuregulin is a neuronal signal that promotes the proliferation and survival and inhibits the differentiation of oligodendrocyte progenitors. *Neuron 1996;* 17: 229-243.

Cole JS, Messing A, Trojanowski JQ, Lee VM. Modulation of axon diameter and neurofilaments by hypomyelinating Schwann cells in transgenic mice. *J.Neurosci. 1994;* 14: 6956-6966.

Coles AJ, Wing MG, Molyneux P et al., Monoclonal antibody treatment exposes three mechanisms underlying the clinical course of multiple sclerosis. *Ann.Neurol. 1999;* 46: 296-304.

Compston A, Coles A. Multiple sclerosis. *Lancet 2002;* 359: 1221-1231.

Compston A. Making progress on the natural history of multiple sclerosis. *Brain 2006;* 129: 561-563.

Confavreux C, Vukusic S, Moreau T, Adeleine P. Relapses and progression of disability in multiple sclerosis. *N.Engl.J.Med. 2000;* 343: 1430-1438.

Confavreux C, Vukusic S. Natural history of multiple sclerosis: a unifying concept. *Brain 2006;* 129: 606-616.

Craner MJ, Lo AC, Black JA, Waxman SG. Abnormal sodium channel distribution in optic nerve axons in a model of inflammatory demyelination. *Brain 2003;* 126: 1552-1561.

Craner MJ, Newcombe J, Black JA, Hartle C, Cuzner ML, Waxman SG. Molecular changes in neurons in multiple sclerosis: altered axonal expression of Nav1.2 and Nav1.6 sodium channels and Na+/Ca2+ exchanger. *Proc.Natl.Acad.Sci.U.S.A 2004;* 101: 8168-8173.

Dai X, Lercher LD, Clinton PM et al., The trophic role of oligodendrocytes in the basal forebrain. *J.Neurosci. 2003;* 23: 5846-5853.

David S, Miller RH, Patel R, Raff MC. Effects of neonatal transection on glial cell development in the rat optic nerve: evidence that the oligodendrocyte-type 2 astrocyte cell lineage depends on axons for its survival. *J.Neurocytol. 1984;* 13: 961-974.

Davie CA, Barker GJ, Webb S et al., Persistent functional deficit in multiple sclerosis and autosomal dominant cerebellar ataxia is associated with axon loss. *Brain 1995;* 118 (Pt 6): 1583-1592.

DeLuca GC, Ebers GC, Esiri MM. Axonal loss in multiple sclerosis: a pathological survey of the corticospinal and sensory tracts. *Brain 2004;* 127: 1009-1018.

DeLuca GC, Williams K, Evangelou N, Ebers GC, Esiri MM. The contribution of demyelination to axonal loss in multiple sclerosis. Brain 2006.

Du Y, Dreyfus CF. Oligodendrocytes as providers of growth factors. *J.Neurosci.Res. 2002;* 68: 647-654.

Dubois-Dalcq M, Ffrench-Constant C, Franklin RJ. Enhancing central nervous system remyelination in multiple sclerosis. *Neuron 2005;* 48: 9-12.

Edgar JM, McLaughlin M, Yool D et al., Oligodendroglial modulation of fast axonal transport in a mouse model of hereditary spastic paraplegia. *J.Cell Biol. 2004;* 166: 121-131.

Elhanany E, Jaffe H, Link WT, Sheeley DM, Gainer H, Pant HC. Identification of endogenously phosphorylated KSP sites in the high-molecular-weight rat neurofilament protein. *J.Neurochem. 1994;* 63: 2324-2335.

Ferguson B, Matyszak MK, Esiri MM, Perry VH. Axonal damage in acute multiple sclerosis lesions. Brain 1997; 120 (Pt 3): 393-399.

Fernandez PA, Tang DG, Cheng L, Prochiantz A, Mudge AW, Raff MC. Evidence that axon-derived neuregulin promotes oligodendrocyte survival in the developing rat optic nerve. *Neuron 2000;* 28: 81-90.

Frohman EM, Racke MK, Raine CS. Multiple sclerosis--the plaque and its pathogenesis. *N.Engl.J.Med. 2006;* 354: 942-955.

Fuchs E, Weber K. Intermediate filaments: structure, dynamics, function, and disease. *Annu.Rev.Biochem. 1994;* 63: 345-382.

Ghatan S, Larner S, Kinoshita Y et al., p38 MAP kinase mediates bax translocation in nitric oxide-induced apoptosis in neurons. *J.Cell Biol. 2000;* 150: 335-347.

Golde S, Chandran S, Brown GC, Compston A. Different pathways for iNOS-mediated toxicity in vitro dependent on neuronal maturation and NMDA receptor expression. *J.Neurochem. 2002;* 82: 269-282.

Goldstein ME, Sternberger NH, Sternberger LA. Phosphorylation protects neurofilaments against proteolysis. *J.Neuroimmunol. 1987;* 14: 149-160.

Grant P, Pant HC. Neurofilament protein synthesis and phosphorylation. *J.Neurocytol. 2000;* 29: 843-872.

Griffiths I, Klugmann M, Anderson T et al., Axonal swellings and degeneration in mice lacking the major proteolipid of myelin. *Science 1998;* 280: 1610-1613.

Jacobs LD, Beck RW, Simon JH et al., Intramuscular interferon beta-1a therapy initiated during a first demyelinating event in multiple sclerosis. CHAMPS Study Group. *N.Engl.J.Med. 2000*; 343: 898-904.

Kapoor R, Davies M, Blaker PA, Hall SM, Smith KJ. Blockers of sodium and calcium entry protect axons from nitric oxide-mediated degeneration. *Ann.Neurol. 2003;* 53: 174-180.

Kappos L. Effect of drugs in secondary disease progression in patients with multiple sclerosis. *Mult.Scler. 2004;* 10 Suppl 1: S46-S54.

Kirkpatrick LL, Witt AS, Payne HR, Shine HD, Brady ST. Changes in microtubule stability and density in myelin-deficient shiverer mouse CNS axons. *J.Neurosci. 2001;* 21: 2288-2297.

Kornek B, Storch MK, Weissert R et al., Multiple sclerosis and chronic autoimmune encephalomyelitis: a comparative quantitative study of axonal injury in active, inactive, and remyelinated lesions. *Am.J.Pathol. 2000;* 157: 267-276.

Kuhlmann T, Lingfeld G, Bitsch A, Schuchardt J, Bruck W. Acute axonal damage in multiple sclerosis is most extensive in early disease stages and decreases over time. *Brain 2002;* 125: 2202-2212.

Lappe-Siefke C, Goebbels S, Gravel M et al., Disruption of Cnp1 uncouples oligodendroglial functions in axonal support and myelination. *Nat.Genet. 2003;* 33: 366-374.

Leary SM, Davie CA, Parker GJ et al., 1H magnetic resonance spectroscopy of normal appearing white matter in primary progressive multiple sclerosis. *J.Neurol. 1999;* 246: 1023-1026.

Leterrier JF, Kas J, Hartwig J, Vegners R, Janmey PA. Mechanical effects of neurofilament cross-bridges. Modulation by phosphorylation, lipids, and interactions with F-actin. *J.Biol.Chem. 1996;* 271: 15687-15694.

Li BS, Veeranna, Gu J, Grant P, Pant HC. Activation of mitogen-activated protein kinases (Erk1 and Erk2) cascade results in phosphorylation of NF-M tail domains in transfected NIH 3T3 cells. *Eur.J.Biochem. 1999;* 262: 211-217.

Li C, Tropak MB, Gerlai R et al., Myelination in the absence of myelin-associated glycoprotein. *Nature 1994;* 369: 747-750.

Lovas G, Szilagyi N, Majtenyi K, Palkovits M, Komoly S. Axonal changes in chronic demyelinated cervical spinal cord plaques. *Brain 2000;* 123 (Pt 2): 308-317.

Lubetzki C, Williams A, Stankoff B. Promoting repair in multiple sclerosis: problems and prospects. Curr.Opin.Neurol. 2005; 18: 237-244.

Lucchinetti C, Bruck W, Parisi J, Scheithauer B, Rodriguez M, Lassmann H. Heterogeneity of multiple sclerosis lesions: implications for the pathogenesis of demyelination. *Ann.Neurol. 2000;* 47: 707-717.

Lucchinetti CF, Bruck W, Rodriguez M, Lassmann H. Distinct patterns of multiple sclerosis pathology indicates heterogeneity on pathogenesis. *Brain Pathol. 1996;* 6: 259-274.

Meyer-Franke A, Kaplan MR, Pfrieger FW, Barres BA. Characterization of the signaling interactions that promote the survival and growth of developing retinal ganglion cells in culture. *Neuron 1995;* 15: 805-819.

Michailov GV, Sereda MW, Brinkmann BG et al., Axonal neuregulin-1 regulates myelin sheath thickness. *Science 2004;* 304: 700-703.

Nixon RA, Paskevich PA, Sihag RK, Thayer CY. Phosphorylation on carboxyl terminus domains of neurofilament proteins in retinal ganglion cell neurons in vivo: influences on regional neurofilament accumulation, interneurofilament spacing, and axon caliber. *J.Cell Biol. 1994;* 126: 1031-1046.

Pang L, Sawada T, Decker SJ, Saltiel AR. Inhibition of MAP kinase kinase blocks the differentiation of PC-12 cells induced by nerve growth factor. *J.Biol.Chem. 1995;* 270: 13585-13588.

Petzold A. Neurofilament phosphoforms: surrogate markers for axonal injury, degeneration and loss. *J.Neurol.Sci. 2005;* 233: 183-198.

Petzold A, Eikelenboom MJ, Keir G et al., Axonal damage accumulates in the progressive phase of multiple sclerosis: three year follow up study. *J.Neurol.Neurosurg.Psychiatry 2005;* 76: 206-211.

Sanchez I, Hassinger L, Sihag RK, Cleveland DW, Mohan P, Nixon RA. Local control of neurofilament accumulation during radial growth of myelinating axons in vivo. Selective role of site-specific phosphorylation. *J.Cell Biol. 2000;* 151: 1013-1024.

Scolding N. Devic's disease and autoantibodies. Lancet Neurol. 2005; 4: 136-137.

Shinar Y, McMorris FA. Developing oligodendroglia express mRNA for insulin-like growth factor-I, a regulator of oligodendrocyte development. *J.Neurosci.Res. 1995;* 42: 516-527.

Smith EJ, Blakemore WF, McDonald WI. Central remyelination restores secure conduction. *Nature 1979;* 280: 395-396.

Smith KJ, Kapoor R, Hall SM, Davies M. Electrically active axons degenerate when exposed to nitric oxide. *Ann.Neurol. 2001;* 49: 470-476.

Smith KJ, Lassmann H. The role of nitric oxide in multiple sclerosis. *Lancet Neurol. 2002;* 1: 232-241.

Strelau J, Unsicker K. GDNF family members and their receptors: expression and functions in two oligodendroglial cell lines representing distinct stages of oligodendroglial development. *Glia 1999;* 26: 291-301.

Trapp BD, Peterson J, Ransohoff RM, Rudick R, Mork S, Bo L. Axonal transection in the lesions of multiple sclerosis. *N.Engl.J.Med. 1998;* 338: 278-285.

Veeranna, Amin ND, Ahn NG et al., Mitogen-activated protein kinases (Erk1,2) phosphorylate Lys-Ser-Pro (KSP) repeats in neurofilament proteins NF-H and NF-M. *J.Neurosci. 1998;* 18: 4008-4021.

Waxman SG, Craner MJ, Black JA. Na+ channel expression along axons in multiple sclerosis and its models. *Trends Pharmacol.Sci. 2004;* 25: 584-591.

Wilkins A, Chandran S, Compston A. A role for oligodendrocyte-derived IGF-1 in trophic support of cortical neurons. *Glia 2001;* 36: 48-57.

Wilkins A, Majed H, Layfield R, Compston A, Chandran S. Oligodendrocytes promote neuronal survival and axonal length by distinct intracellular mechanisms: a novel role for oligodendrocyte-derived glial cell line-derived neurotrophic factor. *J.Neurosci. 2003;* 23: 4967-4974.

Wilkins A, Compston A. Trophic factors attenuate nitric oxide mediated neuronal and axonal injury in vitro: roles and interactions of mitogen-activated protein kinase signalling pathways. *J.Neurochem. 2005;* 92: 1487-1496.

Yin X, Crawford TO, Griffin JW et al., Myelin-associated glycoprotein is a myelin signal that modulates the caliber of myelinated axons. *J.Neurosci. 1998;* 18: 1953-1962.

Yin X, Baek RC, Kirschner DA et al., Evolution of a neuroprotective function of central nervous system myelin. *J.Cell Biol. 2006;* 172: 469-478.

Yool DA, Klugmann M, McLaughlin M et al., Myelin proteolipid proteins promote the interaction of oligodendrocytes and axons. *J.Neurosci.Res. 2001;* 63: 151-164.

Zhao C, Fancy SP, Magy L, Urwin JE, Franklin RJ. Stem cells, progenitors and myelin repair. *J.Anat. 2005;* 207: 251-258.

In: Multiple Sclerosis Research Progress
Editors: H. Schwarz, L. Walter

ISBN: 978-1-60456-570-6
© 2008 Nova Science Publishers, Inc.

Chapter 2

NEUROFILAMENTS AS THE CENTRAL CORE OF AXONAL DAMAGE IN MULTIPLE SCLEROSIS

***Catherine Fressinaud* [1,*] *and Véronique Sazdovitch* [2]**
[1]Neurology Department, University Hospital, Angers Cedex, France
[2]Neuropathology Laboratory, University Hospital Pitié-Salpêtrière, Paris, France

ABSTRACT

Little is known about the proteins involved in axonal damage (AD) which associates with demyelination during multiple sclerosis (MS). Axon transections, amyloid precursor protein accumulation and abnormal expression of the non-phosphorylated form of neurofilaments (NF) have been described. Characterization of AD is a main concern for at least two purposes. First, AD is probably involved in central nervous system (CNS) atrophy, and in patients permanent disability. Second, its impact on remyelination is unknown. Indeed, although neurons are dispensable for oligodendrocytes (OL), the myelinating cells in the CNS, to synthesize myelin-like membranes, neurons enhance this process *in vitro*. Thus, it may be that AD inhibits, in turn, remyelination.

To get insight into these axonal cytoskeleton alterations, we have analyzed by immunohistochemistry 18 chronic plaques from autopsy samples, originating from six MS patients (one progressive, five remitting-progressive forms; mean disease duration: 18.5 years). In comparison to the normal appearing white matter, decreased number of axons immunostained for the three NF subunits, βtubulin, and GAP-43 were - with demyelination and loss of oligodendrocytes (OL) - the hallmarks of plaques, and were extremely severe in 2/3. AD intensity did not correlate with demyelination: although severe demyelination always associated with a 90% decrease in NF+ axons, such severe NF loss also occurred in some plaques despite a moderate demyelination, suggesting it depends too upon other factors. CNP+ and MBP+ OL decreased by the same extent within one plaque, indicating that most OL have reached their final maturation.

* Correspondence to: Dr. Catherine Fressinaud, Neurology Department, UPRES EA 3143, University Hospital, 4 rue Larrey, F49933 Angers Cedex 9, France. E-mail : Catherine.fressinaud@univ-angers.fr; Phone : (33) 2 41 35 46 13; Fax : (33) 2 41 35 35 94

Nevertheless, residual cells show a lower capability to remyelinate axons, since the ratio of MBP+ fibers per OL decreased also.

These results enlarge previous descriptions of cytoskeleton and NF abnormalities in MS, since the expression of the three subunits of NF are decreased, providing evidence that their intimate constituents are impaired. As previously described in animal models, this decrease could lead to axonal atrophy (and slowness of axon potential conduction). Moreover, severe impairment of NF associates with decreased tubulin expression which could result in altered axoplasmic transport. Finally, one can hypothesize that the expression or localization of NF associated proteins (which copurify with NF) could be altered too.

Thus, the body of these results suggests that NF abnormalities are the core of more severe AD than previously hypothesized in MS. Detailing these lesions will help our understanding of permanent disability in MS patients, as well as cues to prevent them. Whether AD might be involved in MS remyelination impairment – which is one of the actual major target of therapeutic hopes such as cell grafts – is under current investigation at the laboratory.

Keywords: axon cytoskeleton, axonal damage, GAP-43, myelin basic protein, neurofilament, oligodendrocyte, tubulin

Abbreviations

AD	axonal damage
CNP	2',3'-cyclic nucleotide 3'-phosphodiesterase
CSF	cerebrospinal fluid
GAP-43	growth associated protein 43
GFAP	glial fibrillary acidic protein
LPC	lysophosphatidyl choline
MBP	myelin basic protein
MS	multiple sclerosis
NF	neurofilament proteins
OL	oligodendrocyte
TUB	tubulin

Introduction

In the course of multiple sclerosis (MS), demyelination is often associated with axonal damage (AD) (Trapp et al., 1998). Nevertheless, the severity of these axonal lesions compared to demyelination, the proteins of the cytoskeleton which are involved, and their mechanisms (Silber and Sharief, 1999), are yet unresolved questions (review in Frohman et al., 2006).

AD is probably involved in central nervous system (CNS) atrophy during MS, and in patient permanent disability (Brück et al., 2002; Losseff et al., 1996), but its impact on remyelination is unknown. Although oligodendrocytes (OL), the myelinating cells in the CNS are able to synthesize and to repair myelin-like membranes *in vitro* even in the absence of neurons (Fressinaud et al., 1990 ; 1996), neurons enhance myelin protein mRNAs and myelin synthesis *in vitro* (Demerens et al., 1996; Macklin et al., 1986). Moreover, axotomy decreases the number of OL precursors in the optic nerve (Barres and Raff, 1993). Thus, it may be that AD in MS inhibits, in turn, remyelination. Therefore it is necessary to clarify the pattern of axonal cytoskeleton lesions, and whether they might impair remyelination since experimentally remyelination can be improved by techniques such as growth factor supply (e. g. Allamargot et al., 2001; Jean et al., 2003) or myelinating cell grafts. Indeed, it has been known for years that myelin has a profound beneficial effect on axonal integrity and that remyelination restores the saltatory conduction of action potentials (review in Zhao et al., 2005). So, in order to remyelinate denuded axons numerous techniques of cell grafts from various origin have been developed including : Schwann cells (e.g., Baron-Van Evercooren et al., 1991; Bachelin et al., 2005), central and olfactory glia (review in Franklin, 2002), adult OL progenitors (Crang et al., 2004), as well as glial precursors derived from embryonic stem cells (Brustle et al., 1999), human embryonic stem cells (Nistor et al., 2005), neural stem cells (review in Cao et al., 2002; Ben-Hur et al., 2003) and bone marrow stromal cells (Akiyama et al., 2002).

Nevertheless, few reports have characterized axonal lesions in MS. Numerous axon transections (Trapp et al., 1998), amyloid precursor protein (APP) accumulation (Ferguson et al., 1997) and abnormal axons expressing the non-phosphorylated form of neurofilaments (NF) (Chang et al., 2002) within active plaques from autopsies, as well as abnormal ubiquitination of axons in the normal appearing white matter (NAWM) (Giordana et al., 2002) have been described. Axonal proteins involved in myelination are also modified : paranodin (which localizes to paranodes when myelination begins) is repressed (Guennoc et al., 2001), and PSA-NCAM, which is believed to inhibit myelination, is reexpressed by some axons in plaques (Charles et al., 2002).

Early in the course of the disease, and even in the NAWM (De Stefano et al., 2001; Narayanan et al., 1997), AD also is suggested by decreased N-acetyl-aspartate peak observed by MRI-spectroscopy. Axonal loss noticed in the NAWM might result from wallerian degeneration of axons transected in the plaques (Evangelou et al., 2000). The increase in the main cytoskeleton proteins (NF L isoform (Lycke et al., 1998), actin and tubulin (Semra et al., 2002), as well as TAU protein (Kapaki et al., 2000) in the cerebrospinal fluid (CSF) of MS patients, correlates to the severity of the disease. Therefore, AD appears to be precocious during MS, nevertheless, its mechanisms are presently unknown: either secondary to the demyelinated status of the axons, and/or due to cytokines released during inflammation (Silber and Sharief, 1999) : OL death and axonal lesions may result from full complement activation (Schwab and McGeer, 2002), and cytotoxic T lymphocytes are able to induce neurite transections *in vitro* (Medana et al., 2001). Bystander killing of neurons by cytotoxic T cells specific for a glial antigen has recently been confirmed in transgenic animals (McPherson et al., 2006).

On the other hand, OL progenitors (Chang et al., 2002; Scolding et al., 1998) and mature OL are either spared, or strongly decreased, depending on plaques even in the same patient, or among authors (e.g., Brück et al., 1994, 2002; Mews et al., 1998; Ozawa et al., 1994; Rodriguez et al., 1993). These conflicting results have not yet received convincing explanations. OL density does not correlate with inflammatory cell infiltration or axonal loss (Lucchinetti et al., 1999). Expression of the anti-apoptotic protein bcl-2 by OL is associated with remyelination, and may contribute to OL preservation in MS (Kuhlmann et al., 1999). Some authors have proposed there could be different histological forms of MS (e.g., Brück et al., 1994; Ozawa et al., 1994). In a large group of actively demyelinating lesions Lucchinetti et al. (2000) identified 4 patterns of demyelination and inflammation, two closely similar with experimental autoimmune encephalomyelitis (EAE), and two suggestive of a primary viral or toxic OL insult. More recently Chang et al. (2002) have observed a high number of OL at a premyelinating stage in some areas of chronic plaques. These cells spread processes contacting demyelinated axons with a dystrophic aspect, suggesting that axons were unsuitable for remyelination. Dystrophic axons have already been described in EAE (Raine and Cross, 1989) or in MS, as well as atrophy (revue in Prineas and McDonald, 1997), but their cytoskeleton has not been characterized, the expression of abnormal non-phosphorylated NF excepted (Chang et al., 2002).

Axonal lesions are better characterized in animal models : in experimental optic neuritis, NF and microtubule loss in some axons, occasional NF ovoid staining, and axonal atrophy are observed (Zhu et al., 1999). Moreover, we have demonstrated that lysophosphatidyl choline (LPC)-induced demyelination in the rat corpus callosum decreases by 50% the axons immunolabelled for the three subunits of NF (NFL, NFM, NFH) and βtubulin (TUB), and that platelet-derived growth factor (PDGF), - which improves remyelination (Allamargot et al., 2001) - , largely reverses these abnormalities (Jean et al., 2002). Since there is no prominent axon loss in this model, this might suggest that demyelination on its own induces AD, and that remyelination alleviates these lesions (Jean et al., 2002). Interestingly we have already observed a similar pattern of cytoskeleton protein alterations in chronic inflammatory demyelinating neuropathy (CIDP, Fressinaud and Jean, 2002), which also shows similarities with MS (Hartung et al., 1999). Therefore, we thought of studying in detail the axonal cytoskeleton proteins in MS, too: a decrease in NF and TUB immunostaining will traduce axonal lesions with more accuracy than the simple counts of transections, whereas an increase in TUB and in GAP-43 will be indicative of a trend to regeneration, since these two proteins are upregulated during development and regeneration (Hoffman et al., 1987 ; Hoffman, 1989).

Materials and Methods

Samples

Brain autopsy samples from six patients suffering histologically confirmed MS (Neuropathology Laboratory, Pr. J.J. Hauw, University Hospital Pitié-Salpêtrière, Paris, France) were analyzed. The samples originated from 3 women and 3 men (mean age : 54.5 ± 11.5 years), 5 were remitting-progressive (RP) forms and one was a primary progressive (PP) form. All patients had EDSS scores > 8.5, and died from infectious or pulmonary complications. Disease duration was in mean 18.5 ± 6 years.

Histology and Immunocytochemistry

Paraffin blocks containing the plaques (three blocks per brain) were cut in serial sections (7 μm thick) which were used for luxol-fast blue (LFB)-phloxin-hematein staining and immunohistochemistry. Chronic plaques were recognized by the absence of LFB-positive inclusions in macrophages (Giordana et al., 2002; Prineas and McDonald, 1997).

The cytoskeleton components were labelled with antibodies raised against each of the three neurofilament subunits (light, medium, and heavy chain: NFL, NFM, NFH, Sigma) and βtubulin (TUB, Sigma). The axons were also stained with anti-growth associated protein antibody (GAP-43, Biotrend, Köln, Germany). Antibodies raised against myelin basic protein (MBP, Dako, Trappes, France), myelin proteolipid (PLP, gift of Dr. E. Trifilieff (Trifilieff et al., 1986)), 2',3'-cyclic nucleotide 3'-phosphodiesterase (CNP, Sigma Immunochemicals, St Louis, MO), and glial fibrillary acidic protein (GFAP, Dako) were used to label myelin and oligodendrocytes (MBP, PLP, CNP), or astrocytes (GFAP), respectively. Biotinylated secondary antibodies (Amersham, Les Ulis, France) and avidin-biotin-horseradish peroxydase H complex (Vectastain ABC kit, Vector Laboratories, Burlingame, CA) were used for 3,3'-diaminobenzidine tetrahydrochloride (Sigma) staining. Sections were counterstained with hematein. Procedures were performed as previously described (Fressinaud et al., 2002, 2005; Jean et al., 2002).

Cell and Fiber Counting

Axonal transections (i.e., interruption of fiber continuity) in plaques were semi-quantitatively estimated on LFB-stained sections and, depending on the number of preserved fibers, expressed as mild (-25%), moderate (-50%) or severe (-100%, i.e., virtually all the axons were transected) compared to the adjacent normal appearing white matter (NAWM).

Immunolabelled cells (OL and astrocytes) and the entire cell population (defined by nucleus staining with hematein) were counted in the totality of standardized microscopic fields defined by an ocular morphometric grid using a X 100 objective. Similarly the number of immunolabelled fibers for myelin antibodies, and the number of axons stained for antibodies to the cytoskeleton, or to GAP-43, were counted per optic field. All these measurements were performed in five optic fields within each of the plaques, and in 5 optic fields in the adjacent NAWM. In this latter the fibers were so dense that it precluded a perfectly accurate counting of myelinated fibers and of axons labelled for cytoskeleton components, these values represent therefore rather a precise estimation and are slightly underevaluated (i.e., between two counts in the same field differences from 10 to less than 50 fibers were encountered for a total number of 400 to 10^3 fibers, depending on the antibody used, and on the anatomic localization). Results were first expressed as mean ± SD of counts per optic field within the plaque, or in the NAWM. To allow comparison between plaques counts were subsequently expressed as percentage of variation compared to the NAWM.

Comparison of mean counting between plaques and NAWM employed Mann and Whitney test.

RESULTS

Since MS is primary characterized by demyelination we first characterized plaques on the basis of myelin and OL loss.

Demyelination and Oligodendrocyte Loss

Demyelination (Figures 1A and 2A), loss of OL, and axonal lesions (transections as well as decreased immunostaining for cytoskeleton proteins) (Figures 2B, 3, and 4) were the hallmarks of plaques, excepted in one block (4*2) where OL number was modestly increased (non significant). Comparison of the number of CNP+ and MBP+ cells within one plaque gave similar results (Figure 2A), as well as that of PLP+ OL (not shown), indicating that most OL have reached their final maturation stage and were therefore susceptible to remyelinate axons (attempts to use anti-MOG antibody were unsuccessful). OL number (CNP+, PLP+, and MBP+ cells per optic field) was generally decreased compared to the NAWM ($\alpha < 1\%$, Mann and Whitney test).

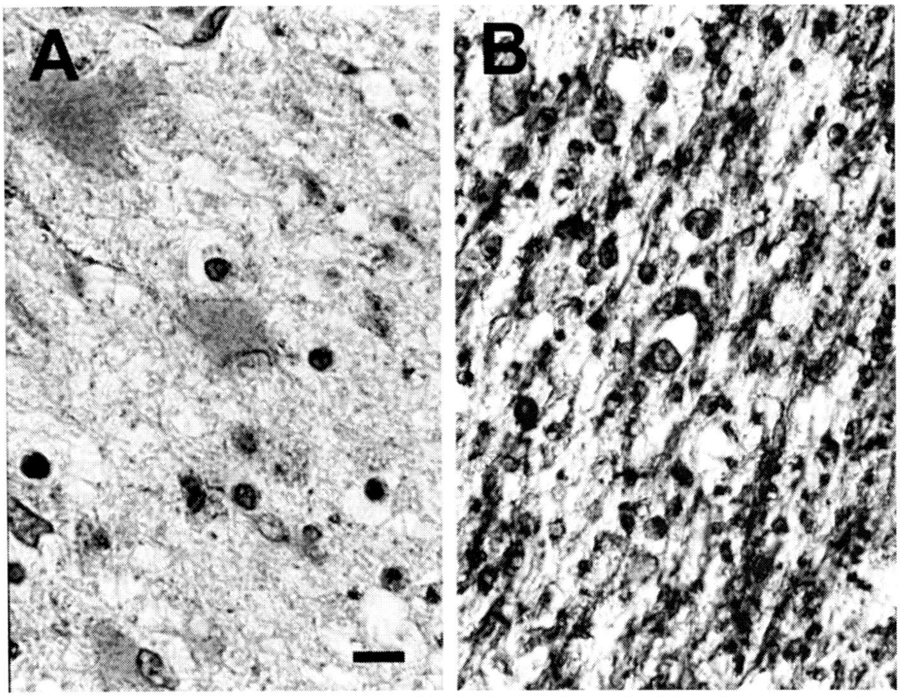

Figure 1. Immunohistochemistry of MS plaque (block PP6*1 (**A**)) and of the adjacent normal appearing white matter (**B**), with anti-MBP antibody (peroxydase, hematein counterstain). Despite preservation of quite numerous axons, note complete demyelination in (**A**) compared to (**B**), whereas some MBP+ oligodendrocytes are still present in the plaque. Bar = 10 µm.

Since the lack of remyelination could simply result from this decrease in mature (MBP+) OL, we also calculated the capability of theses cells to myelinate axons: i.e., the ratio of myelinated fibers per OL (MBP+ fibers / MBP+ OL). This demonstrated that residual cells showed a lower capability to myelinate axons, - or axons were unproper for remyelination - , since this ratio also decreased, by 37 to 100%, compared to the NAWM (Figures 1A and 2A). Moreover, it was also decreased in block 4*2, despite the increased number of MBP+ OL.

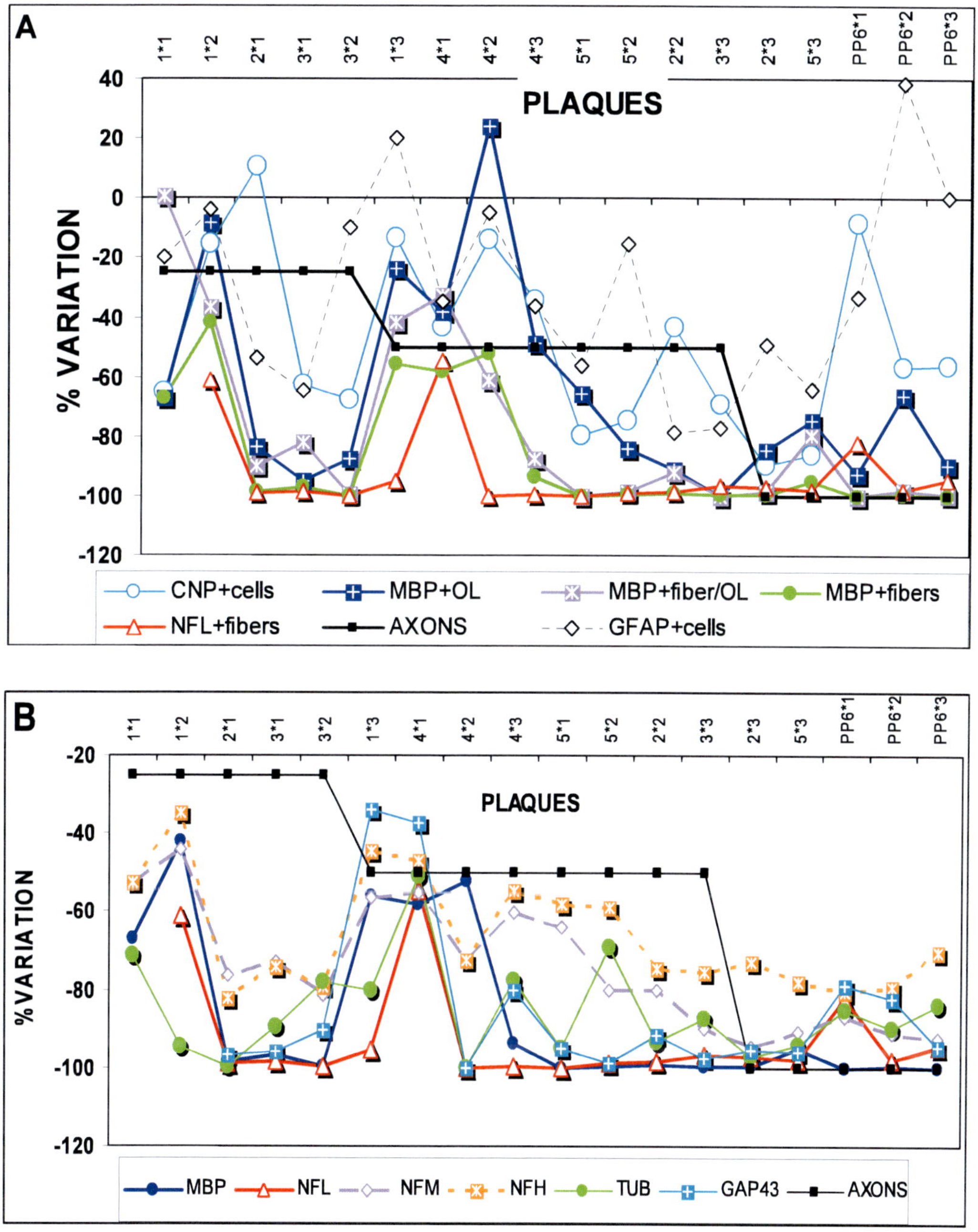

Figure 2. (Continues.)

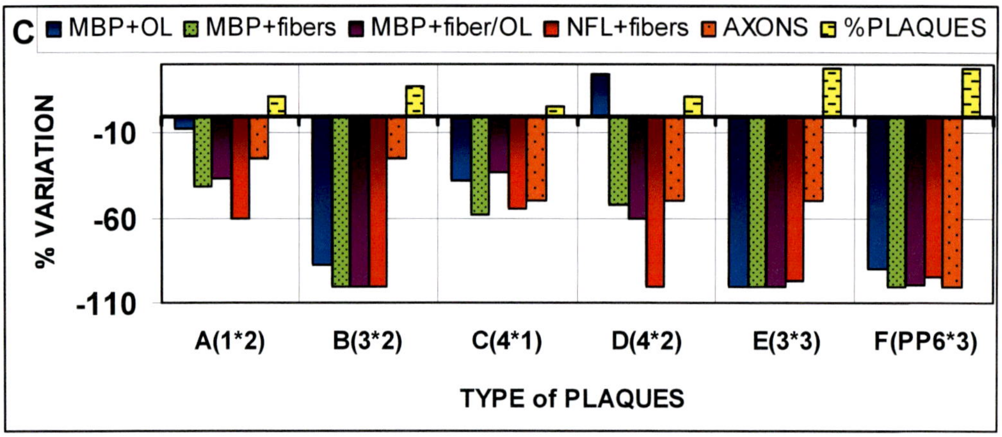

Figure 2. Results of immunohistochemistry for each of the 18 plaques (**A**, **B**) (patient number * block number, PP denotes the primary progressive form) presented by order of increasing axonal transections that were semi-quantitatively expressed as mild (-25%), moderate (-50%) or severe (-100%). (**A**) Labelled cells and/or fibers for antibodies directed against myelin (CNP, MBP, and the ratio of MBP+ fibers per MBP+ oligodendrocytes) are compared to astrocytes (GFAP+ cells), and to NFL. Results are expressed as percentage of variation compared to the adjacent normal appearing white matter (NAWM, mean of counts in 5 optic fields). (**B**) Results of axonal cytoskeleton immunohistochemistry compared to demyelination for each of the 18 plaques that have been analyzed (mean counts of 5 optic fields). (**C**) Classification of MS plaques in 6 types (A-F) by increasing severity of axonal transections, demyelination (MBP+ fibers), and NFL loss. Results are expressed as percentage of variation compared to the adjacent NAWM. One representative example of each type of plaque (number of patient * number of sample) is presented. The percentage of plaques of each type is given (yellow bars).

Astrocytic Gliosis

Astrocyte morphology was modified with a rigid aspect and an increase in the number of spine-like processes, suggestive of astrocytic gliosis (not shown). In most cases, however, the number of GFAP+ cells decreased (non significant) (Figure 2A) in the plaques compared to the NAWM. Rather an "astrocytic line" could be delineated at the edges of the plaques : rows of astrocytes were often delimiting the plaques (not shown).

Axonal Cytoskeleton Damage

Axonal lesions comprised axonal transections, which were constant (Figure 2B). Moreover, in 13/18 plaques (72%), they were semi-quantitatively quantified as moderate (50% axon loss) or severe (nearly 100% axon loss). Dystrophic axons were sometimes encountered (Figure 3C), but we did not observe ovoid.

Even in residual axons without transactions the cytoskeleton was frequently affected: these axons (and the continuity of the axonal cylinder) were still observable with the hematein counterstain, but they were not labelled by the different antibodies (NFL, NFM, NFH, TUB, and GAP-43) used (Figures 3 and 4). It was striking that all the cytoskeleton proteins, as well as GAP-43, were strongly decreased (> 50%) compared to the NAWM (α < 1%, Mann and

Whitney test), although NFM and NFH were less severely affected than NFL, TUB and GAP-43 (Figure 2B). Indeed, TUB and GAP-43 were generally decreased by 80% (TUB) to 100% (GAP-43), in 2 lesions excepted (blocks 1*3 and 4*1), and correlated with NFL decrease, indicating that there was no trend to regeneration.

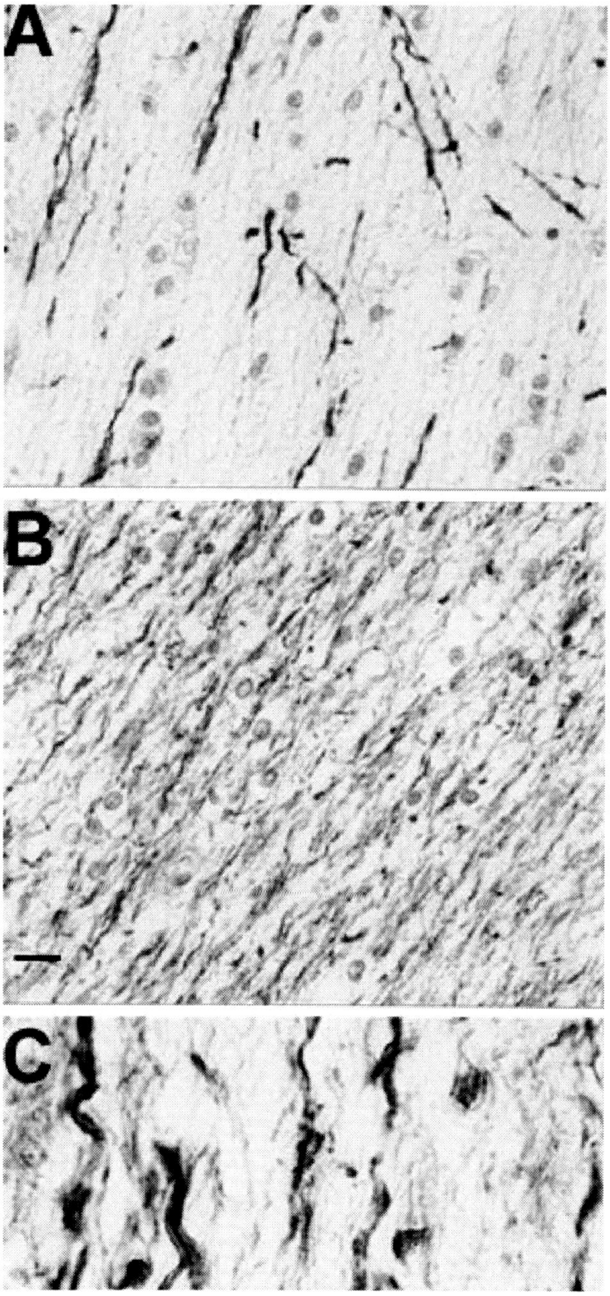

Figure 3. Immunohistochemistry of MS plaque (block 4*2) (**A** and **C**) and of the adjacent normal appearing white matter (**B**), with anti-NFH antibody (peroxydase, hematein counterstain). Despite preservation of some axons, note nearly complete loss of neurofilament immunostaining in (**A** and **C**) compared to (**B**), while still labelled axons appear tortuous and dystrophic in the plaque at higher magnification (**C**). Bar = 20 μm in **A** and **B**, 10 μm in **C**.

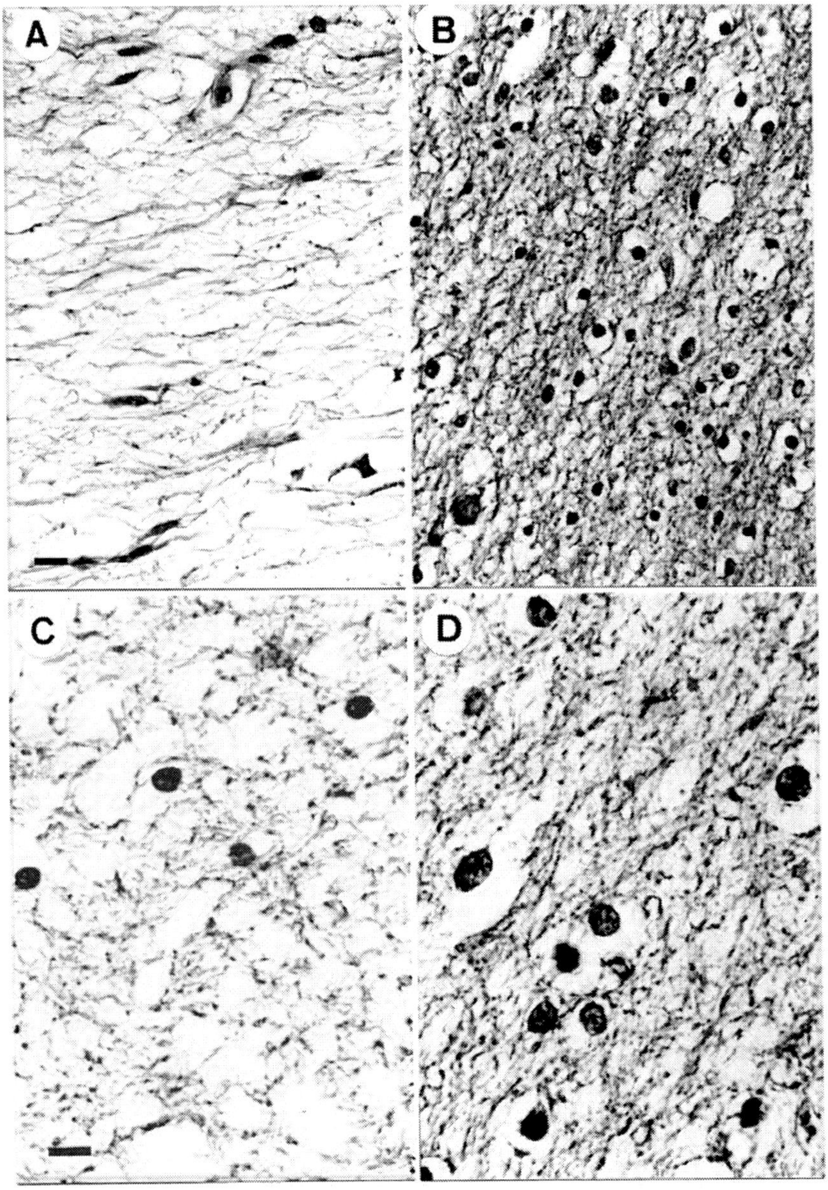

Figure 4. Immunohistochemistry of MS plaque (block 4*2) (**A** and **C**) and of the adjacent normal appearing white matter (**B** and **D**), with anti-β tubulin (**A**, **B**) and anti-GAP-43 (**C**, **D**) antibodies (peroxydase, hematein counterstain). Despite preservation of some axons, note nearly complete loss of axon immunostaining in (**A** and **C**) compared to (**B** and **D**) respectively. Bar = 20 μm in **A** and **B**, 10 μm in **C** and **D**.

Major axonal transections were, unsurprisingly, associated with severe defects in axonal cytoskeleton proteins immunolabelling (> 80%) (as observed in case PP6) (Figure 2B). Nevertheless, these defects also occurred in association with more moderate axonal transections. For example the number of fibers immunostained for NFL decreased by 98% in blocks 2*1, 3*1, and 3*2, whereas axon loss was only estimated by 25% in these 3 lesions. This indicated that axon loss did not account for the extent of decreased immunostaining in cytoskeletal proteins, and that additional AD was present in these cases.

Thus, the only PP form (case PP6) included in this study coincided with the most severe pattern of axonal transections, loss of staining for axonal cytoskeleton proteins, and complete demyelination. Nevertheless this pattern of complete destruction could also be observed in RP forms (blocks 5*3 and 2*3 for example, Figure 2B). So, in these latter several types of profiles could be delineated (Figure 2A, 2B): i) either moderate (block 4*1) or severe (block 5*3) destruction of myelin and axons that were correlated, ii) or, dissociation between severe demyelination and cytoskeleton lesions contrasting with moderate axonal loss (blocks 4*3, 5*1, and 5*2). Conversely, a strong decrease in NFL immunolabelling and pronounced axonal transections (block 1*3) could be observed, despite relative preservation of myelin. In some plaques (1*3, and 4*2) also moderate demyelination and axonal transections contrasted with nearly complete loss in NFL immunostaining. Finally, severe demyelination was always associated with major cytoskeleton abnormalities, but these latter could also accompanied more moderate demyelination.

Classification of Plaques

Depending on axonal transections, NFL loss and demyelination, we classified plaques in six representative types of lesions by increasing severity (Figure 2C): i) mild axonal transections associated with either moderate demyelination and moderate NFL loss (2 lesions, 11.11%, type A), or with severe demyelination and severe NFL loss (three lesions, 16.67%, type B); ii) moderate axonal transections associated with either moderate demyelination and moderate NFL loss (one lesion, 5.56%, type C), or moderate demyelination and severe NFL loss (two lesions, 11.11%, type D), or severe demyelination and severe NFL loss (five lesions, 27.78%, type E). This type E was therefore the most frequent encountered together with the last type (more than 55% in all), i.e.: iii) severe axonal transections associated with severe demyelination and severe NFL loss (5 lesions, 27.78%, type F), this type corresponded to the three lesions of the PP form, and to two of RP forms.

Mean duration of disease was not significantly different between the PP form (20 years) and RP forms (18.2 ± 6.5 years). Nevertheless, it was striking that complete axonal transections and demyelination were observed in only 2/15 (13 %) of RP forms, versus 3/3 plaques of the PP form; moreover this type of lesion concerned only 1/3 plaques of these two RP forms. In all, 10/15 (67 %) plaques of RP forms comprised complete demyelination and NFL loss, two (13%) with major axonal transections (type F), five (33%) with moderate axonal transections (type E), and 3 (20%) with mild axonal transections (type B). Although there was a relative homogeneity of lesions for one given patient, i.e., at least 2/3 plaques of the same type were observed in 5/6 cases (83%), there was as many type of lesions as of patients.

In search for correlations with the classification of active plaques (Lassmann, 2002), we observed that most of these chronic plaques had sharp edges (types I, II and IV of Lassmann), and 10/18 (55 %), including the totality (three blocks) of three cases were very well delimited (not shown). Only five plaques were centred by a vessel. Vessels were generally numerous within the plaques, with perivascular infiltration in one case (RP1*) only, and often distributed at random. In addition to the five plaques with at least one central vessel, three elongated plaques had venules centring their extremities. There was no correlation between these parameters and the intensity of myelin or axonal destruction.

DISCUSSION

Although the histology of MS has been described long ago, relatively few studies have analyzed in parallel the fate of myelin, OL and of axons. The severity of demyelination and of axonal cytoskeleton damage that we observed in these chronic lesions was striking since 72% showed complete demyelination and NFL loss. This appears a severe evolution for a disease duration that was in mean < 19 years in our cases, with a mean age of apparition of clinical signs of 32 years. Although our study is based on a small number of cases, it is important to note, despite a mean duration of disease similar to that of RP forms, that the more severe immunohistochemical pattern of axon destruction and demyelination (major axonal transections and complete MBP and NFL loss) corresponded mostly to the only PP form studied - since it was observed in 3/3 lesions analysed, a pattern which was never observed in the totality of the plaques for one case in RP forms - . Nevertheless, this PP form represented 16% of our cases, which is in the range of frequency (10-15%) of PP forms generally reported (e.g., Ingle et al., 2002; McDonnell and Hawkins, 2002). This in accordance with the literature pointing out the severity of MS PP forms (Bashir and Whitaker, 1999; Brück et al., 2002; McDonnell and Hawkins, 2002; Thompson et al., 1997). It has been reported that cerebrospinal fluid from patients with PP – but not those with RP forms – of MS induces neuron apoptosis *in vitro* (Øren et al., 2001). Such a neurotoxic factor could explain, at least partly, the severity of these forms, while primary OL degeneration, - which seems to be the hallmark of MS PP forms (Brück et al., 2002) - , might explain the failure of remyelination. The report of Wolswijk (2000) has already emphasized the decrease in mature and immature OL in chronic progressive MS, our results showing a 70-90% decrease in OL in case PP6 is in accordance with this observation.

Our results also strengthen the notion that axonal lesions (transections as well as decrease in cytoskeleton proteins expression) are a prominent feature of MS plaques, since they were constantly observed, and, most frequently (15/18, 83% with complete NFL loss), moderate or severe. AD therefore is not limited to acute lesions where it has been reported too (Bitsch et al., 2000). This is akin to the data of Mews et al. (1998) who found an average of 55-65% reduction in axon density. We have already observed very similar alterations of the cytoskeleton (without fiber transections) in experimental studies, where they appeared consecutive to demyelination itself, and improved during remyelination (Jean et al., 2002). In MS, nevertheless, and as shown here, they may occur even in the presence of moderate demyelination (5/18, 28%; and five out of five plaques with moderate demyelination). Given the early axonal degeneration observed for example in double mutant *plp-/-mag-/-* which lacks compact myelin (Uschkureit et al., 2000), this result is not surprising : sustained demyelination - even mild - in MS might be deleterious for axons. Nevertheless, the lack of congruence between the severity of demyelination and that of axonal impairment in our study could suggest that this latter depends also on other factors, such as cytotoxic cytokines, reactive oxygen and NO species, or glutamate (revue in Silber and Sharief, 1999). The fact that axonal injury is, at least in part, independent of demyelination has already been reported (Bitsch et al., 2000).

Profound decrease (around 100%) in immunolabelling for the axonal proteins studied (NF, TUB, and GAP-43) was observed in some of our cases even in the absence of severe axonal loss (-25%) indicating that : first, decreased number of immunostained axons is not only due to fiber loss, and , second, that additional AD appears more extended than previously reported. Similarly, we have previously demonstrated that LPC-induced demyelination induces decreased NF expression in rat corpus callosum despite the lack of significant fiber loss in this model (Allamargot et al., 2001), and that remyelination alleviates these lesions (Jean et al., 2002).

The precise nature of the axonal cytoskeleton lesions in MS also has not been described to our knowledge; most authors have used only the SMI-32 antibody (e.g., Chang et al., 2002; Trapp et al., 1998), which labels the abnormal non-phosphorylated forms of NF, or anti-amyloid antibody (Bitsch et al., 2000; Ferguson et al., 1997) and, for axonal transections excepted, only qualitative studies of axonal damage have been reported. It was remarkable that all the cytoskeleton proteins (the 3 NF subunits, and TUB) that we have studied were affected, although NFL and TUB were more severely decreased. Pronounced decrease in TUB and GAP-43 immunolabelling indicated that there was no trend to regeneration since these two proteins are upregulated during it (Hoffman et al., 1987; Hoffman, 1989). As TUB and GAP-43 decreased in parallel to NFL, this confirms that these proteins can be used as valuable markers of AD during MS, as previously reported by CSF studies (Lycke et al., 1998).

Since NF are major determinants of axonal caliber (Hoffmann et al., 1987; Eyer and Peterson, 1994), the strong decrease in NF we observed in plaques could have severe consequences on axonal architecture as well as metabolism, and might also account for axonal atrophy, which is a recognized feature of MS plaques (Prineas and McDonald, 1997). Decreased NF expression may arise from demyelination, as demonstrated in our LPC model (Jean et al., 2002). Indeed, during development axon ensheathment by OL processes induces local accumulation of NF, triggering thereby full axon radial growth (Sanchez et al., 1996; Windebank et al., 1985). Conversely, the lack of remyelination might be explained, at least in part, if axons do not reach the adequate caliber (Dyck et al., 1984; Hoffmann et al., 1987).

Nevertheless, other results from our group suggest that the lack of NF might not be per see the origin of the remyelination defect in MS. Indeed, we have observed in NFH-lacZ transgenic mice – which lack axonal NF (Eyer and Peterson, 1994) and show constitutive CNS (as well as PNS) axonal atrophy – that remyelination proceeds as well as in their wild-type littermates after LPC-induced demyelination of the corpus callosum (Jean and Fressinaud, 2003). This demonstrates that, at least, constitutive lack of axonal NF does not impair CNS remyelination. This model also confirmed that demyelination induces axonal atrophy in wild-type mice, a phenomenon known to slow down axon potential conduction (review in Sargent, 1992), and thus able to impair proper function of axons leading finally to disability.

Moreover, the profound decrease in TUB that we observed in MS also could result in altered axoplasmic transport along microtubules (review in Hammerschlag and Brady, 1989), which is likely to impair even more axon metabolism. Indeed, altered axoplasmic transport might affect too proteins involved in axon-glia interactions, and especially in myelination, providing thereby additional perturbations to the repair process. Such molecules comprise for example neuregulins which are expressed by axons and promote OL development and myelination (review in Falls, 2003) and which have been implicated in MS physiopathology (e. g. Cannella et al., 1999, Viehover et al., 2001).

In order to get insights into the putative impact of decreased NF expression observed in MS on the remyelination process, we have started another experimental approach to determine the effects of NF and/or their associated proteins on OL fate. Although these neurocytoskeletal elements are physiologically intracytoplasmic, they could either mediate a signal to OL through their binding to transmembrane proteins, or they could be present in the extracellular space following an axonal lesion and modulate remyelination. Indeed, during NF purification procedures (Fasani et al., 2004) numerous proteins copurify with NF (e.g., STOP proteins (Letournel et al., 2003)). Preliminary results reveal that *in vitro* adult rat brain NF enriched fractions, obtained by successive purification steps, significantly enhanced OL progenitor proliferation as well as their differentiation and maturation into OL (Fressinaud et al., 2006), compared to controls, in pure OL secondary cultures grown in chemically defined medium (Fressinaud et al., 1990; Fressinaud, 2005). Molecules responsible for these effects are currently under investigation at the laboratory, and their expression will be assessed in MS plaques in search for correlations with demyelination and AD.

Thus, the body of these results strengthen the hypothesis that severe impairment of axonal cytoskeleton, involving NF, TUB, (and/or their associated proteins) that we observed in MS plaques might have severe consequences on both axon metabolism, and remyelination, and finally create a vicious circle leading to patient permanent disability.

It is also important to draw comparisons between AD in MS and other pathological or experimental conditions. This pattern of decreased NF and TUB immunostaining in MS is similar to what we have observed in: i) toxic demyelination of the CNS in rodents - where there is no prominent fiber loss - (Jean et al., 2002); and ii) in cases of chronic inflammatory demyelinating neuropathy (CIDP) presenting with fiber loss (Fressinaud and Jean, 2002). On the contrary, in axonopathies of unknown aetiology, and in necrotizing vasculitis of the peripheral nervous system (Fressinaud et al., 2002, 2003, 2005), TUB increased and was inversely correlated with fiber density and NFL, which decreased. Thus, primary demyelination involving either the CNS (MS, LPC-induced demyelination) or the PNS (CIDP), whatever its mechanisms may be (probably autoimmune : MS and CIDP, or toxic : LPC-induced), could result in the same axonal cytoskeleton alterations, which are clearly distinct from those encountered in primary axonal pathologies. In a therapeutic perspective, it is important to note also that remyelination alleviates acute axonal damage in our toxic model (Jean et al., 2002).

In most of our MS cases OL were strongly decreased (over 50%) in the plaques, compared to the NAWM, in accordance with previous studies (Brück et al., 1994; Mews et al., 1998; Ozawa et al., 1994; Rodriguez et al., 1993). Recent *in vitro* studies using LPC toxicity have demonstrated that the repetition of attacks is deleterious for cells of the OL lineage (Fressinaud, 2005). Thus, it is likely that repeated relapses account – at least in part - for OL loss in RP MS plaques. Subsequently, this decrease in myelinating cells could represent one of the main factors limiting remyelination. From this point of view, our study in MS does not match with that of Chang et al. (2002), since we observed a number of MBP+ cells (as well as of PLP+ cells) that was generally equivalent to that of CNP+ cells in plaques. This demonstrates that nearly all surviving OL had reached their final maturation stage, and were therefore susceptible to remyelinate axons. Also, Chang et al. (2002) reported that "many" premyelinating OL extended processes contacting axons without myelination; in our cases we did not detect such type of cells. This apparent discrepancy could be due to the technique used by these authors (microwave pretreatment, thickness of sections > 30μm, and > 5 days incubation with primary antibody) that differs from ours.

Our data introduce a new notion concerning OL in MS plaques : we observed in addition that in all cases the capability of OL to remyelinate axons was decreased by 37 to 100%, even in the block where the number of OL was slightly increased. Indeed, fibers unlabelled for MBP (and counterstained by hematein), with a normal aspect (i.e.,not dystrophic) and crossing the plaques could be observed in most cases, indicating that this lack of remyelination was unlikely due – at least in these cases – to axonal dystrophy or transections. Such disturbances of the myelinating function of OL have been reported (Rodriguez et al., 1993). To explain the failure of remyelination in MS this mechanism of OL dysfunction could represent an alternative to the hypothesis of a causal axonal impairment proposed by Chang et al. (2002), based on their observations of the association between OL processes and abnormal axons. Though, our results might in turn be compatible with the assumption that, despite their normal morphology, axons are unproper for remyelination, for example as a consequence of paranodin repression (Guennoc et al., 2001), or PSA-N CAM reexpression (Charles et al., 2002). Nevertheless, it cannot be concluded yet that these latters are sufficient to explain on their own the lack of remyelination. As demonstrated and discussed above, NF loss (resulting in axonal atrophy), decreased OL density, and impairment of OL capability to synthesize new membranes after several attacks, are also likely involved in the failure of myelin repair.

We were unable to match up the histology of these chronic lesions with the classification of active plaques (Lassmann, 2002), which could have explained the variabilty of histological damage depending on the situation of fibers compared to vessels. This could be due to the repetition of attacks in these chronic lesions, modifying the architecture of the plaques, for example by extension of the process to additional vessels.

As described previously (revue in Prineas and McDonald, 1997), astrocytic gliosis was not a prominent feature of MS plaques. Rather, as reported in EAE (Matsumoto et al., 1992), an "astrocytic limit" could be delineated at the edges of the plaques Although astrocytes are involved in the course of CNS repair (e.g., Matsumoto et al., 1992; Ridet et al., 1997; Westenbroek et al., 1998), and might protect newly generated OL by internalization (Wu and Raine, 1992), or terminal axonal sprouts by PSA-N CAM+ ensheathment (Dusart et al., 1999), there is little evidence from our results to draw conclusions about their role. At least it can be assumed that astrocyte density did not increase in the plaques in our cases. Nevertheless, the peculiar arrangement of their processes could be sufficient to modify significantly, even on the only architectural point of view, the environment of injured axons and damaged myelin sheathes.

CONCLUSION

Pronounced AD, involving all the major cytoskeleton components (NF and TUB) together with GAP-43, is now characterized in MS chronic plaques, and it occurs in nearly ¾ of the lesions, even in the absence of major axonal transactions or demyelination. This strengthens the hypothesis that axon injury also depends upon other components (probably involved in the inflammatory process). Comparative analyses reveal that NFL appears as a good marker of AD, since TUB and GAP-43 decrease to the same extent. Depending on the severity of axonal and myelin damage, we have identified several types of lesions, confirming the heterogeneity of pathological patterns among patients (Brück et al., 1994, 2002;

Lassmann, 2002; Ozawa et al., 1994), and the lack of correlation between demyelination and AD (Bitsch et al., 2000). In addition, this study emphasizes the facts that OL are decreased and that their capability to synthesize new myelin sheathes is impaired.

Although our study should be confirmed by analyses of a greater number of samples, its results bring arguments favouring the utilization, early in the course of MS, of efficient therapeutics that will take into account the axonal as well as the myelin components of plaques. From this point of view it is relevant to remember that, experimentally, growth factor supply alleviates, at least partly, both these demyelinating and axonal lesions (Jean et al., 2002).

Acknowledgments

Supported by a grant (PHRC 21-01) from the University Hospital of Angers to CF. We thank the neurologists from the Departments of Neurology from Pitié-Salpêtrière Hospital for their help in collecting clinical data, and Ms. I. Viau and C. Dumez for skillful technical assistance.

References

Akiyama Y, Radtke C, Kocsis JD. (2002). Remyelination of the rat spinal cord by transplantation of identified bone marrow stromal cells. *J Neurosci.* 22, 8823-8830.

Allamargot, C., Pouplard-Barthelaix, A., Fressinaud, C. (2001). A single intracerebral injection of platelet-derived growth factor (PDGF) accelerates the rate of remyelination in vivo. *Brain Res.* 918, 28-39.

Bachelin C, Lachapelle F, Girard C, Moissonnier P, Serguera-Lagache C et al., (2005). Efficient myelin repair in the macaque spinal cord by autologous grafts of Schwann cells. *Brain 1*28, 540-549.

Baron-Van Evercooren, A., Gansmüller, A., Clerin, E., Gumpel, M. (1991). Visualization of Schwann cells transplanted in a demyelinated lesion of the adult mouse spinal cord. *Neurosci. Lett.* 131, 241-244.

Barres, B.A., Raff, M.C. (1993). Proliferation of oligodendrocyte precursor cells depends on electrical activity in axons. *Nature* 361, 258-260.

Bashir, K., Whitaker, J.N. (1999). Clinical and laboratory features of primary progressive and secondary progressive MS. *Neurology* 53, 765-771.

Ben-Hur T, Einstein O, Mizrachi-Kol R, Ben-Menachem O, Reinhartz E et al., (2003). Transplanted multipotential neural precursor cells migrate into the inflamed whitte matter in response to experimental autoimmune encephalomyelitis. *Glia* 41, 73-80.

Bitsch, A., Schuchardt, J., Bunkowski, S., Kuhlmann, T., Bruck, W. (2000). Acute axonal injury in multiple sclerosis. Correlation with demyelination and inflammation. *Brain* 123, 1174-1183.

Brück, W., Schmied, M., Suchanek, G., Brück, Y., Breitschopf, H., Poser, S., Piddlesden, S., Lassmann, H. (1994). Oligodendrocytes in the early course of multiple sclerosis. *Ann. Neurol.* 35, 65-73.

Brück, W., Lucchinetti, C., Lassmann, H. (2002). The pathology of primary progressive multiple sclerosis. *Mult. Scler.* 8, 93-97.

Brustle O, Jones KN, Learish RD, Karram K, Choudhary K et al., (1999). Embryonic stem cell-derived glial precursors : a source of myelinating transplants. *Science* 285, 650-651.

Cannella B, Pitt D, Marchionni M, Raine CS. (1999). Neuregulin and erbB receptor expression in normal and diseased human white matter. *J Neuroimmunol* 100, 233-242.

Cao Q, Benton RL, Whittemore SR. (2002). Stem cell repair of central nervous system injury. *J Neurosci Res* 68, 501-510.

Chang, A., Tourtelotte, W.W., Rudick, R., Trapp, B.D. (2002). Premyelinating oligodendrocytes in chronic lesions of multiple sclerosis. *N. Engl. J. Med.* 346, 165-173.

Charles, P., Reynolds, R., Seilhean, D., Rougon, G., Aigrot, M.S., Neizgoda, A., Zalc, B., Lubetzki, C. (2002). Re-expression of PSA-NCAM by demyelinated axons : an inhibitor of remyelination in multiple sclerosis ? *Brain* 125, 1972-1979.

Crang AJ, Gilson JM, Li WW, Blakemore WF. (2004). The remyelinating potential and in vitro differentiation of MOG-expressing oligodendrocyte precursors isolated from the adult rat CNS. *Eur J Neurosci* 20, 1445-1460.

Demerens, C., Stankoff, B., Anglade, P., Allinquant, B., Couraud, F., Zalc, B., Lubetzki, C. (1996). Induction of myelination in the central nervous system by electrical activity. *Proc. Natl. Acad. Sci. USA* 93, 9887-9892.

De Stefano, N., Narayanan, S., Francis, G.S., Arnaoutelis, R., Tartaglia, M.C., Antel, J.P., Matthews, P.M., Arnold, D.L. (2001). Evidence of axonal damage in the early stages of multiple sclerosis and its relevance to disability. *Arch. Neurol.* 58, 65-70.

Dusart, I., Morel, M.P., Wehrle, R., Sotelo, C. (1999). Late axonal sprouting of injured Purkinje cells and its temporal correlation with permissive changes in the glial scar. *J. Comp. Neurol.* 408, 399-418.

Dyck, P.J., Nukada, H., Lais, A.C., Karnes, J.L. (1984). Permanent axotomy: A model of chronic neuronal degeneration preceded by axonal atrophy, myelin remodeling and degeneration. In: Dyck PJ, Thomas PK, Lambert EH, Bunge R. (Eds), *Peripheral neuropathy, Saunders, Philadelphia*, pp. 666-690.

Evangelou, N., Konz, D., Esiri, M.M., Smith., S, Palace, J., Matthews, P.M. (2000). Regional axonal loss in the corpus callosum correlates with cerebral white matter lesion volume and distribution in multiple sclerosis. *Brain* 123, 1845-1849.

Eyer J, Peterson A. (1994). Neurofilament-deficient axons and perikaryal aggregates in viable transgenic mice expressing a neurofilament-b-galactosidase fusion protein. *Neuron* 12:389-405.

Falls DL. (2003). Neuregulins: functions, forms, and signalling strategies. *Exp Cell Res* 284, 14-30.

Fasani F, Bocquet A, Robert P, Peterson A, Eyer J. (2004). The amount of neurofilaments aggregated in the cell body is controlled by their increased sensitivity to trypsin-like proteases. *J Cell Sci* 117:861-869.

Ferguson, B., Matyszak, M.K., Esiri, M.M., Perry, V.H. (1997). Axonal damage in acute multiple sclerosis lesions. *Brain* 120, 393-399.

Franklin RJM, 2002). Remyelination of the demyelinated CNS: the case for and against transplantation of central, peripheral and olfactory glia. *Brain Res Bull* 57, 827-832.

Fressinaud, C., Vallat, J.M., Rigaud, M., Cassagne, C., Labourdette, G., Sarliève, L.L. (1990). Investigation of myelination in vitro: polar lipid content and fatty acid composition of myelinating oligodendrocytes in rat oligodendrocyte cultures. *Neurochem. Int.* 16, 27-39.

Fressinaud, C., Vallat, J.M., Pouplard-Barthelaix, A. (1996). Platelet-derived growth factor partly prevents chemically induced oligodendrocyte death and improves myelin-like membranes repair in vitro. *Glia* 16, 40-50.

Fressinaud, C., Jean, I. (2002). Polyradiculonévrites inflammatoires chroniques et cytosquelette axonal : données morphométriques et immunocytochimiques. *Rev. Neurol.* (Paris) 158, 713-718.

Fressinaud, C., Vigneron, I., Letournel, F., Nicolas, G., Jean, I., Dubas F. (2002). Cytoskeleton abnormalities in axonopathies of unknown aetiology: correlations with morphometry. *J. Neurol. Sci.* 196, 53-61.

Fressinaud, C., Jean, I., Dubas, F. (2003). Vascularites nécrosantes du système nerveux périphérique : comparaison des anomalies du cytosquelette axonal avec d'autres types de neuropathies. *Rev. Neurol.* (Paris) 159, 293-299.

Fressinaud, C. (2005). Repeated injuries dramatically affect cells of the oligodendrocyte lineage : effects of PDGF and NT-3 in vitro. *Glia* 49, 555-566.

Fressinaud, C., Jean, I., Dubas, F. (2005). Modifications des neurofilaments et des microtubules axonaux en fonction du mécanisme lésionnel : étude pathologique et expérimentale. *Rev. Neurol.* (Paris) 161, 55-60.

Fressinaud, C., Berges, R., Bocquet, A., Eyer, J. (2006). Neurofilament associated proteins specifically alter oligodendrocyte development in vitro : relevance for MS. *J. Neurochem.*, 2006, 96 (Suppl. 1), Abstract PTW08-2 p. 133.

Frohman EM, Racke MK, Raine CS. (2006). Multiple sclerosis – The plaque and its pathogenesis. *N Engl J Med* 354, 942-955.

Giordana, M.T., Richiardi, P., Trevisan, E., Boghi, A., Palmucci, L. (2002). Abnormal ubiquitination of axons in normally myelinated white matter in multiple sclerosis brain. *Neuropathol. Appl. Neurobiol.* 28, 35-41.

Guennoc, A.M., Stankoff, B., Barbin, G., Zalc, B., Lubetzki, C. (2001). Rôle de la paranodine dans la myélinisation du SNC. *Rev. Neurol.* (Paris) 157, suppl 3, 2S51 abstract F13.

Hammerschlag R, Brady ST. (1989). Axonal transport and the neuronal cytoskeleton. In: *Basic neurochemistry.* Siegel G, Agranoff B, Albert RW, Molinoff P (Eds), Raven Press, New York, pp. 457-478.

Hartung, H.P., Ritz, M.F., Steck, A.J. (1999). Eléments de neuro-immunologie. In: . Steck, A.J., coordinator, Bogousslavsky, J., Léger, J.M., Mas, J.L., (Eds), *Affections démyélinisantes. Neuroimmunologie et clinique. Traité de neurologie.* Doin, Rueil-Malmaison, pp. 35-60.

Hoffman, P.N., Cleveland, D.W., Griffin, J.W., Landes, P.N., Cowan, N.J., Price, D.L. (1987). *Neurofilament gene expression : a major determinant of axonal caliber.* Proc. Natl. Acad. Sci. USA 84, 3472-3476.

Hoffman, P.N. (1989). Expression of GAP-43, a rapidly transported growth-associated protein and class II beta tubulin, a slowly transported cytoskeletal protein, are coordinated in regenerating neurons. *J. Neurosci.* 9, 893-897.

Ingle, G.T., Thompson, A.J., Miller, D.H. (2002). Magnetic resonance imaging in primary progressive multiple sclerosis. *J. Rehabil. Res.* Dev. 39, 261-271.

Jean, I., Allamargot, C., Barthelaix-Pouplard, A., Fressinaud, C. (2002). Axonal lesions and PDGF-enhanced remyelination in the rat corpus callosum after lysolecithin demyelination. *Neuroreport* 13, 627-631.

Jean I, Fressinaud C. (2003). Spontaneous central nervous system remyelination is not altered in NFH-lacZ transgenic mice after chemical demyelination. *J Neurosci Res* 73:54-60.

Jean, I., Lavialle, C., Barthelaix-Pouplard, A., Fressinaud, C. (2003). Neurotrophin-3 specifically increases mature oligodendrocyte population and enhances remyelination after chemical demyelination of adult rat CNS. *Brain Res.* 972, 110-118.

Kapaki, E., Paraskevas, G.P., Michalopoulou, M., Kilidireas, K. (2000). Increased cerebrospinal fluid tau protein in multiple sclerosis. *Eur. Neurol.* 43, 228-232.

Kuhlmann, T., Lucchinetti, C., Zettl, U.K., Bitsch, A., Lassmann, H., Brück, W. (1999). Bcl-2 expressing oligodendrocytes in multiple sclerosis lesions. *Glia* 28, 34-39.

Lassmann, H., 2002. Mechanisms of demyelination and tissue destruction in multiple sclerosis. *Clin. Neurol. Neurosurg.* 104, 168-171.

Letournel F, Bocquet A, Dubas F, Barthelaix A, Eyer J. (2003). Stable tubule only polypeptides (STOP) proteins co-aggregate with spheroid neurofilaments in amyotrohic lateral sclerosis. *J Neuropathol Exp Neurol* 62:1211-1219.

Losseff, N.A., Webb, S.L., O'Riordan, J.I., Page, R., Wang, L., Barker, G.J., Tofts, P.S., McDonald, W.I., Miller, D.H., Thompson, A.J. (1996). Spinal cord atrophy and disability in multiple sclerosis. A new reproductible and sensitive MRI method with potential to monitor disease progression. *Brain* 119, 701-708.

Lucchinetti, C., Brück, W., Parisi, J., Scheithauer, B., Rodriguez, M., Lassmann, H. (1999). A quantitative analysis of oligodendrocytes in multiple sclerosis. A study of 113 cases. *Brain* 122, 2279-2295.

Lucchinetti, C., Brück, W., Parisi, J., Scheithauer, B., Rodriguez, M., Lassmann, H. (2000). Heterogeneity of multiple sclerosis lesions: implications for the pathogenesis of demyelination. *Ann. Neurol.* 47, 707-717.

Lycke, J.N., Karlsson, J.E., Andersen, O., Rosengren, L.E. (1998). Neurofilament protein in cerebrospinal fluid: a potential marker of activity in multiple scerosis. J. Neurol. Neurosurg. *Psychiatry* 64, 402-404.

Macklin, W.B., Weill, C.L., Deininger, P.L. (1986). Expression of myelin proteolipid and myelin basic protein mRNAs in culture cells. *J. Neurosci. Res.* 16, 203-217.

McDonnell, G.V., Hawkins, S.A. (2002). Primary progressive multiple sclerosis : increasing clarity but many unanswered questions. *J. Neurol. Sci.* 199, 1-15.

McPherson SW, Heuss ND, Roehrich H, Gregerson DS. (2006). Bystander killing of neurons by cytotoxic T cells specific for a glial antigen. Glia 53, 457-466.

Matsumoto, Y., Ohmori, K., Fujiwara, M. (1992). Microglial and astroglial reactions to inflammatory lesions of experimental autoimmune encephalomyelitis in the rat central nervous system. *J. Neuroimmunol.* 37, 23-33.

Medana, I., Martinic, M.A., Wekerle, H., Neumann, H. (2001). Tansection of major histocompatibility complex class I-induced neuritis by cytotoxic T lymphocytes. *Am. J. Pathol.* 159, 809-815.

Mews, I., Bergmann, M., Bunkowski, S., Gulotta, F., Brück, W. (1998). Oligodendrocyte and axon pathology in clinically silent multiple sclerosis lesions. *Mult. Scler.* 4, 55-62.

Narayanan, S., Fu, L., Pioro, E., De Stefano, N., Collins, D.L., Francis, G.S., Antel J.P., Matthews, P.M., Arnold, D.L. (1997). Imaging of axonal damage in multiple sclerosis: spatial distribution of magnetic resonance imaging lesions. *Ann. Neurol.* 41, 385-391.

Nistor GI, Totoiu MO, Haque N, Carpenter MK, Kierstead HS. (2005). Human embryonic stem cells differentiate into oligodendrocytes in high purity and myelinate after spinal cord transplantation. *Glia* 49, 385-396.

Øren, A., White, L.R., Aasly, J. (2001). Apoptosis in neurons exposed to cerebrospinal fluid from patients with multiple sclerosis or acute polyradiculoneuropathy. *J. Neurol. Sci.* 186, 31-36.

Ozawa, K., Suchanek, G., Breitschopf, H., Brück, W., Budka, H., Jellinger, K., Lassmann, H. (1994). Patterns of oligodendroglia pathology in multiple sclerosis. *Brain* 117, 1311-1322.

Prineas, J.W., McDonald, W.I. (1997). Demyelinating diseases. In: Graham DI, Lantos PL. (Eds), *Greenfield's neuropathology,* Arnold, London, pp. 813-896.

Raine, C.S., Cross ,A.H. (1989). Axonal dystrophy as a consequence of long-term demyelination. Lab. Invest. 60, 714-725.

Ridet, J.L., Malhotra, S.K., Privat, A., Gage, F.H., 1997). *Reactive astrocytes: cellular and molecular cues to biological function.* TINS 20, 570-577.

Rodriguez, M., Scheithauer, B.W., Forbes, G., Kelly, P. (1993). Oligodendrocyte injury is an early event in lesions of multiple sclerosis. *Mayo Clin. Proc.* 68, 627-636.

Sanchez, I., Hassinger, L., Paskevich, P.A., Shine, H.D., Nixon, R.A. (1996). Oligodendroglia regulate the regional expansion of axon caliber and local accumulation of neurofilaments during development independently of myelin formation. . *Neurosci.* 16, 5095-5105.

Sargent PB, 1992). Signalisation électrique. In : *Introduction à la neurobiologie moléculaire.* Hall ZW (Ed), Flammarion, Paris, pp. 33-80.

Schwab, C., McGeer, P.L. (2002). Complement activated C4d immunoreactive oligodendrocytes delineate small cortical plaques in multiple sclerosis. *Exp. Neurol.* 174, 81-88.

Scolding, N., Franklin, R., Stevens, S., Heldin, C.H., Compston, A., Newcombe, J. (1998). Oligodendrocyte progenitors are present in the normal adult human CNS and in the lesions of multiple sclerosis. *Brain* 121, 2221-2228.

Semra, Y.K., Seidi, O.A., Sharief, M.K. (2002). Heightened intrathecal release of axonal cytoskeletal proteins in multiple sclerosis is associated with progressive disease and clinical disability. *J. Neuroimmunol.* 122, 132-139.

Silber, E., Sharief, M.K. (1999). Axonal degeneration in the pathogenesis of multiple sclerosis. *J. Neurol. Sci.* 170, 11-18.

Thompson, A.J., Polman, C.H., Miller, D.H., McDonald, W.I., Brochet, B., Filippi, M., Montalban, X., De Sa, J. (1997). Primary progressive multiple sclerosis. *Brain* 120, 1085-1096.

Trapp, B.D., Peterson, J., Ransohof, R.M., Rudick, R., Mörk, S., Bö, L. (1998). Axonal transection in the lesions of multiple sclerosis. *N. Engl. J. Med.* 338, 278-285.

Trifilieff, E., Luu, B., Nussbaum, J.L., Roussel, G., Espinosa de los Monteros, A., Sabatier, J.M., Van Rietschoten, J. (1986). A specific immunological probe for the major myelin proteolipid. Confirmation of a deletion in DM 20. *FEBS Lett.* 198, 235-239.

Uschkureit, T., Spörkel, O., Stracke, J., Büssow, H., Stoffel, W. (2000). Early onset of axonal degeneration in double (plp-/-mag-/-) and hypomyelinosis in triple (plp-/-mbp-/-mag-/-) mutant mice. *J. Neurosci.* 20, 5225-5233.

Viehover A, Miller RH, Park SK, Fischbach G, Vartanian T. (2001). Neuregulin: an oligodendrocyte growth factor absent in active multiple sclerosis lesions. *Dev Neurosci* 23, 377-386.

Westenbroek, R.E., Bausch, S.B., Lin, R.C., Franck, J.E., Noebels, J.L., Catterall, W.A. (1998). Upregulation of L-type Ca2+ channels in reactive astrocytes after brain injury, hypomyelination, and ischemia. *J. Neurosci.* 18, 2321-2334.

Windebank, A.J., Wood, P., Bunge, R.P., Dyck, P.J. (1985). Myelination determines the caliber of dorsal root ganglion neurons in culture. *J. Neurosci.* 5, 1563-1569.

Wu, E., Raine, C.S. (1992). Multiple sclerosis, interactions between oligodendrocytes and hypertrophic astrocytes and their occurrence in other, nondemyelinating conditions. *Lab. Invest.* 67, 88-99.

Zhao C, Fancy SPJ, Magy L, Urwin JE, Franklin RJM. (2005. Stem cells, progenitors and myelin repair. *J Anat* 207, 251-258.

Zhu, B., Moore, G.R.W., Zwimpfer, T.J., Kastrukoff, L.F., Dyer, J.K., Steeves, J.D., Paty, D.W., Cynader, M.S. (1999). Axonal cytoskeleton changes in experimental optic neutitis. *Brain Res.* 824, 204-217.

In: Multiple Sclerosis Research Progress
Editors: H. Schwarz, L. Walter
ISBN: 978-1-60456-570-6
© 2008 Nova Science Publishers, Inc.

Chapter 3

FURTHER EVIDENCE FOR THE PSYCHOMETRIC PROPERTIES OF THE ABBREVIATED LATE-LIFE FUNCTION AND DISABILITY INSTRUMENT IN INDIVIDUALS WITH MULTIPLE SCLEROSIS

Robert W. Motl and Edward McAuley
Department of Kinesiology and Community Health
University of Illinois at Urbana-Champaign, IL USA

ABSTRACT

The measurement of functional limitations and disability in individuals with multiple sclerosis (MS) has been plagued by definitional ambiguity and measurement limitations. The abbreviated Late Life-Function and Disability Inventory (LL-FDI) was recently developed based on accepted definitions of functional limitations and disability, and has been preliminarily supported as having good measurement properties in individuals with MS. This study further examined the structural and external aspects of score validity for the LL-FDI in individuals with MS. Individuals with MS completed the LL-FDI and measures of physical activity, walking mobility and neurological impairment. Structural aspects of score validity for the LL-FDI were established using confirmatory factor analysis (CFA). The CFA confirmed the existence of two factors of personal and social aspects of disability for the disability frequency and limitations subscales of the LL-FDI, and three factors of upper extremity function, basic lower extremity function, and advanced lower extremity function for the functional limitations subscale of the LL-FDI. External aspects of score validity for the LL-FDI were established based on expected differences in mean scores between individuals with relapsing-remitting MS and primary and secondary progressive MS and examination of the pattern of correlations between mean scores with the measures of physical activity, walking mobility, and neurological impairment. Our results further support the structural and external aspects of score validity for the LL-FDI in individuals with MS, and we recommend that future researchers use this scale when measuring functional limitations and disability in this population.

INTRODUCTION

Multiple sclerosis (MS) is a chronic and progressive disease of the central nervous system (National Multiple Sclerosis Society [NMSS], 2005) and functional limitations and disability are likely consequences of the disease. MS involves a presumed attack by the immune system of the myelin sheath that surrounds the axons of neurons in the central nervous system. This results in demyelination and transection of axons and interferes with the salutatory conduction of action potentials. The interference with conduction of action potentials results in multiple symptoms including loss of function and feeling in limbs, fatigue, loss of balance and coordination, pain, cognitive dysfunction, and depression (NMSS, 2005; Lublin, 2005). Ultimately, the symptoms lead to functional limitations and disability. For example, 50% of individuals will require the use of an aid for walking (i.e., reach an Expanded Disability Status Scale score of 6.0) and 10% will require a wheelchair within 15 years after the onset of MS (Weinshenker et al., 1989; Runmarker and Anderson, 1993). Nearly 90% of individuals will have functional limitations and disability within 25 years after the onset of MS (Frohman, Racke, and van den Noort, 2000).

Nevertheless, current measures of functional limitations and disability are inadequate and lack sensitivity for detecting the types of change experienced by people with MS (Coulthard-Morris, 2000). This is, in part, attributable to the very nature of the disease (Rudick et. al., 1996) were the clinical course of MS is unpredictable and varies among individuals and across time (Coulthard-Morris, 2000). Another contributing factor is that existing measures have not been developed within an established model of physical disablement that provides sound operational definitions of functional limitations and disability.

The measurement of functional limitations and disability in MS might benefit by consideration of the disablement process. Based on Nagi's (1976) model of the disablement process and Verbrugge and Jette's (1994) operational definitions, Guralnik and Ferrucci (2003) differentiated functional limitations and disability as two important components of the disablement process. Functional limitations can be described as an individual's reduced capacity to carry out activities that are relevant for effective community living such as walking, lifting, climbing, reaching, and handling everyday objects. Disability can be described as an individual's inability for performing socially defined roles and tasks within a sociocultural and physical environment (Nagi, 1976).

The original (Jette et al., 2002) and abbreviated (McAuley, Konopack, Motl, Rosengren, and Morris, 2005) versions of the Late-Life Function and Disability Instrument (LL-FDI) represent methodological advancements in the measurement of functional limitations and disability. The original LL-FDI was developed based on the disablement process and consists of three components, namely Functional Limitations, Disability Frequency, and Disability Limitations. The original LL-FDI was developed using a sample of 150 adults aged 60 years and older, and contained a comprehensive battery of items that avoided problems such as ceiling and floor effects by spreading items across a broad range of activities (Jette et al., 2002). We recently revised and abbreviated the LL-FDI based on an examination of its psychometric properties and construct validity in a sample of older women (McAuley et al., 2005). This abbreviated version of the LL-FDI had an acceptable 15-item solution for the Functional Limitations component and an acceptable 8-item solution for both the Disability Frequency and Disability Limitation components. The Functional Limitations component consisted of three subscales of advanced lower extremity function, basic lower extremity function, and upper extremity function. The Disability Frequency and Disability Limitations components each consisted of two subscales of performing social and personal role activities. This abbreviated instrument demonstrated high correlations with the original LL-FDI scales. Construct validity for the abbreviated LL-FDI was supported based on correlations with measures of physical function, body composition, and physical activity. The abbreviated LL-FDI appears to be an effective instrument for assessing function and disability in older women, although continued determination of its structural and construct aspects of validity is recommended in similar and different populations.

The content and conceptual underpinnings of the LL-FDI make it amenable for use with diseased populations, including individuals with MS. We previously provided preliminary evidence for the structural and external aspects of score validity of the LL-FDI in individuals with MS (Motl, Snook, Gosney, and McAuley, 2008). Structural aspects of score validity were examined using confirmatory factor analysis (CFA). The CFA supported the existence of two factors of personal and social aspects of disability for the disability frequency and limitations subscales of the LL-FDI, and three factors of upper extremity function, basic lower extremity function, and advanced lower extremity function for the functional limitations subscale of the LL-FDI. External aspects of score validity for the LL-FDI were based on expected differences in mean scores between individuals with relapsing-remitting MS and primary and secondary progressive MS and examination of the pattern of correlations between mean scores with the measures of physical activity, neurological impairment, walking mobility, and quality of life.

This study further examined the structural and external aspects of score validity for the abbreviated LL-FDI in individuals with MS. We initially confirmed the structural validity of the Disability and Functional Limitations components of the abbreviated LL-FDI using standard covariance modeling procedures and confirmatory factor analysis. After confirming the structural validity, we examined the reliability of the scales using estimates of internal consistency derived using Cronbach's coefficient alpha. We then tested the external aspects of score validity for the abbreviated LL-FDI based on known-groups comparisons of scores between individuals with relapsing-remitting and progressive forms of MS and correlations with measures of physical activity, walking mobility, and neurological impairment.

METHODS

Participants

The sample consisted of individuals with MS who were members of three chapters of the MS society using (a) research announcements mailed to past study participants, (b) advertisements placed in each Chapter's *MS Connection* quarterly publication, and (c) email messages that were distributed to all registered members of the Chapters. Those interested in participation were asked to contact the research team through either e-mail or telephone, and collect calls were encouraged and accepted from those interested in participating and living outside the local calling area. This initial contact was followed-up by a phone call from a member of the research team who described the study and its procedures, answered all questions, and conducted a brief screening interview. The screening criteria involved (a) having an established definite diagnosis of MS, (b) being relapse free in the last 30 days, and (c) being ambulatory with minimal assistance. The definite diagnosis was confirmed based on completion of a form-letter by the participant's neurologist. Individuals were relapse free as we suspect that physical activity would be substantially reduced during and immediately after such an episode. Ambulatory with minimal assistance was defined as being able to walk with or without a cane, but excludes those using a wheelchair or motorized cart.

There were 511 individuals who were contacted about participation in this study, and 387 of those individuals underwent screening. Of those who were screened, there were 27 individuals who did not satisfy our inclusion criteria and 16 individuals who declined participation. We sent an informed consent document and verification letter to the remaining 344 individuals, and the forms were returned by 300 of the 344 individuals. Of those who returned the forms, 8 did not continue with participation and reasons for lack of participation are unknown. The final convenience sample consisted of 292 individuals with MS. The sample consisted of 245 women and 47 men, and 246 were diagnosed with relapsing-remitting MS (RRMS), 12 were diagnosed with primary progressive MS (PPMS), and 34 were diagnosed with secondary progressive MS (SPMS). The mean age of the sample was 48.0 years (*SD* = 10.3, range = 20 – 69 years) and the mean duration, defined as time since definite diagnosis, of MS was 10.3 years (*SD* = 7.9, range = 1 – 35 years). The sample was mostly Caucasian (94%), married (68%), employed (53%), and educated (28% had some college education & 57.7% were college graduates) with a median annual household income of greater than $40,000 (67.7%).

Measures

LL-FDI

The abbreviated LL-FDI (McAuley et al., 2005) is a multidimensional measure of function and disability with good psychometric properties (Jette et al., 2002). The function component of the abbreviated LL-FDI contains a 15-item self-report measure of functional limitations (limitations in a person's ability to do discrete actions or activities) that correspond with advance lower extremity function, basic lower extremity function, and upper extremity function. An example item for the advance lower extremity function was "How much difficulty do you have with going up and down a flight of stairs outside, without using a handrail?". An example item for the basic lower extremity function was "How much difficulty do you have using a step stool to reach into a high cabinet?". An example item for the upper extremity function was "How much difficulty do you have unscrewing the lid off a previously unopened jar without using any devices?". The 15-items were rated on a 5-point scale of 1 (none) and 5 (cannot do) and were reverse-scored and then averaged to form composite measures of advance lower extremity function, basic lower extremity function, and upper extremity function with higher scores representing better functioning; scores for each subscale range between 5 and 25.

The disability component of the abbreviated LL-FDI contains an 8-item measure of disability frequency (i.e., frequency of performing socially-defined tasks) and an 8-item measure of disability limitations (i.e., limitations with performing socially-defined tasks) that both correspond with social and personal components of disability. An example item for the social component of disability limitations was "To what extent do you feel limited in visiting friends and family in their homes?". An example item for the personal component of disability limitations was "To what extent do you feel limited in taking care of your own personal care needs?". The 8-items for the disability frequency component were rated on a 5-point scale of 1 (never) and 5 (very often). The 8-items for the disability limitation component were rated on a 5-point scale of 1 (not at all) and 5 (completely). The items on both scales were reverse-scored and then averaged to form composite measures of social and personal components of disability frequency and limitations with higher scores representing less disability; scores for each subscale range between 4 and 20.

Physical Activity

We measured physical activity using the ActiGraph single-axis accelerometer (model 7164 version, Health One Technology, Fort Walton Beach, FL). We have previously provided validity evidence for this measure of physical activity in individuals with MS (Gosney, Scott, Snook, and Motl, 2007; Motl, Snook, McAuley, and Scott, 2006). This accelerometer contains a single, vertical axis piezoelectric bender element that generates an electrical signal proportional to the force acting on it. Acceleration detection ranges in magnitude from 0.05 - 3.2 Gs and the frequency response ranges from 0.25 - 2.5 Hz. Motion outside normal human movements is rejected by a band-pass filter. The acceleration/deceleration signal is digitized by an analog-to-digital converter and numerically integrated over a pre-programmed epoch interval yielding activity counts. Hence, activity counts are a summation of accelerations measured during a cycle period that is established along with start time during an initialization phase. The counts represent a quantitative measure of activity over time, and are linearly related to the intensity of a participant's physical activity during a cycle period. The cycle period, or epoch, can range from 1 second to 10 minutes, and in this study was set to be 1 minute. Each accelerometer was checked for accuracy using manufacturer-recommended hardware and software and calibrated, if necessary. We further checked each accelerometer for accuracy using a walking test (15 minutes of walking at 80 $m \cdot min^{-1}$ on a treadmill). All accelerometers were accurate based on manufacturer recommended criteria and our walking test. Participants recorded the time the units were worn in a log on a daily basis.

Walking Mobility

We measured walking mobility using the Patient Determined Disease Steps (PDDS) scale (Hadjimichael, Kerns, Rizzo, Cutter, and Vollmer, 2007). The PDDS is a self-report questionnaire that contains a single item for measuring self-reported mobility-disability using an 8-level ordinal scale. Scores from the PDDS are linearly and strongly related with physician-administered EDSS scores ($r = .93$; Hadjimichael et al., 2007).

Neurological Impairment

Neurological impairment was measured by the Symptom Inventory (SI; Schwartz, Vollmer, and Lee, 1999). The SI is composed of 99 items that are rated using a 5-point scale based on the severity of symptoms experienced in the past month. The items reflect six subscales (correlated with localization of brain lesions) of Visual, Left Hemisphere, Right Hemisphere, Brain Stem and Cerebellum, Spinal Cord, and Nonlocalized Symptoms. The SI is scored by computing the mean item score for each subscale and summing the subscale mean scores for a total score. This scale has good evidence for its internal consistency and test-retest reliability and preliminary evidence for its construct, discriminant, and incremental validity as a measure of neurological impairment in MS (Marrie and Goldman, in press; Schwartz et al., 1999). The internal consistency of the items on the SI in the present study was .97 based on coefficient alpha.

Procedure

The procedure for this study was approved by the University of Illinois at Urbana-Champaign Institutional Review Board, and all participants provided written informed consent. As part of a longitudinal investigation of physical activity and quality of life, the participants completed a battery of questionnaires that included the abbreviated LL-FDI, PDDS, and SI, and wore the accelerometer during the waking hours (i.e., the moment upon getting out of bed in the morning through the moment of getting into bed in the evening), except while showering, bathing, and swimming, for a seven-day period. The participants recorded the time that the accelerometer was worn on a log, and this was verified by inspection of the minute-by-minute accelerometer data. Participants received $20 and a pedometer as remuneration after completing the measures and wearing the accelerometer.

Data Analysis

Factorial Validity

The fit of measurement models for the components of the abbreviated LL-FDI was examined using confirmatory factor analysis with maximum likelihood estimation in LISREL 8.50. The fit of the measurement models was evaluated based on the chi-square statistic, standardized root mean square residual (SRMR), and comparative fit index (CFI). The chi-square statistic assesses perfect fit of the model to the data (Bollen, 1989). The SRMR is the average of the standardized residuals between the specified and obtained variance-covariance matrices. The SRMR should be less than .08 to indicate good model fit (Hu and Bentler, 1999). The CFI is an incremental fit index, and tests the proportionate improvement in fit by comparing the target model to a baseline model with no correlations among observed variables (Bentler, 1990). CFI values approximating 0.90 and 0.95 were indicative of acceptable and good model-data fit, respectively (Bentler, 1990; Hu and Bentler, 1999).

Internal Consistency

After confirming the factorial validity, we next examined the internal consistency of subscale and overall composite scores from the disability and functional components of the abbreviated LL-FDI. The analysis of internal consistency was undertaken using Cronbach's coefficient alpha and SPSS for Windows 15.0.

Construct Validity

The first method of establishing the construct validity of scores on the abbreviated LL-FDI involved comparisons of disability and function subscale scores between individuals with RRMS and those with PPMS/SPMS. This was accomplished using a one-way (Groups: RRMS vs. PPMS/SPMS) multivariate analysis of variance (MANOVA) on scores from function and disability frequency and limitation components of the abbreviated LL-FDI. The multivariate main effect was decomposed using univariate *F*-ratios and the magnitude of the group differences were expressed using Cohen's *d*. The second method of examining the construct validity of scores on the abbreviated LL-FDI involved examining correlations with measures of physical activity (Accelerometer), walking mobility (PDDS), and neurological impairment (SI). This was accomplished using Pearson product-moment correlations computed between scores from the function and disability component of the abbreviated version of the LL-FDI with scores from the Accelerometer, PDDS, and SI. Both the MANOVA and correlation analysis were undertaken using SPSS for Windows 15.0.

RESULTS

Factorial Validity

Disability Component – Frequency Items

We initially confirmed the fit of two, correlated factors consisting of personal and social roles for the 8-item Disability, Frequency component of the abbreviated LL-FDI. The model represented a good fit for the data ($\chi^2 = 28.23$, df = 19, $p = .08$, SRMR = .05, CFI = 0.99). All factor loadings were statistically significant, and the items and factor loadings for the model are presented in table 1. The standardized correlation between the personal and social role factors was statistically significant ($\varphi = 0.48$).

Table 1. Standardized factor loadings for the items on the Disability-Frequency and Disability-Limitation scales of the LL-FDI

Items	Disability, Frequency		Disability, Limitations	
	Personal	Social	Personal	Social
Take care of local errands	.71		.81	
Prepare meals	.68		.77	
Take care of personal care needs	.43		.65	
Take care of household business	.42		.59	
Go out to public places		.68		.78
Visit friends		.74		.81
Travel out of town		.58		.79
Invite family and friends into home		.65		.71

Disability Component – Limitation Items

We then confirmed the fit of two, correlated factors consisting of personal and social roles for the 8-item Disability, Limitation component of the abbreviated LL-FDI. This model represented an excellent fit for the data (χ^2 = 42.91, df = 19, p = .001, SRMR = .03, CFI = 0.98). All factor loadings were statistically significant, and the items and factor loadings for the final model are presented in table 1. The standardized correlation between the personal and social role factors was statistically significant (φ = 0.84).

Function Component

We finally confirmed the fit of three, correlated factors consisting of advanced lower body extremity function, basic lower body extremity function, and upper extremity function with correlated uniqueness between items 14 and 15 and items 3 and 4 on the basic lower body extremity and upper extremity function factors, respectively, for the 15-item Function component of the abbreviated LL-FDI. This model provided an improved and good fit for the data (χ^2 = 203.79, df = 85, p = .0001, SRMR = .05, CFI = 0.95). All factor loadings were statistically significant, and the items and factor loadings for the final model are presented in table 2. There were statistically significant standardized correlations between advanced lower body extremity function and basic lower body extremity function (φ = .81), advanced lower body extremity function and upper extremity function (φ = .61), and basic lower body extremity function and upper extremity function (φ = .71).

Table 2. Standardized factor loadings for the items on the Functional Limitations scales of the LL-FDI

Items	ALEF	BLEF	UEF
Go up and down 1 flight, no rails	.85		
Carry while climb stairs	.87		
Walk 1 mile with rests	.76		
Go up and down 3 flights inside	.74		
Run one-half mile	.68		
Get into and out of car		.71	
Bend over from a standing position		.72	
Pick up a kitchen chair		.77	
On and off a step stool		.76	
Walk around one floor of home		.69	
Pour from a large pitcher			.85
Remove wrapping with hands only			.80
Hold full glass of water in 1 hand			.65
Use common utensils			.68
Unscrew lid without assistive device			.66

Note. ALEF = advanced lower extremity function. BLEF = basic lower extremity function. UEF = upper extremity function.

Internal Consistency

The estimates of internal consistency were acceptable for the personal (α = .64) and social (α = .76) roles subscale scores and composite score (α = .74) for the 8-item Disability, Frequency component of the abbreviated LL-FDI. The estimates of internal consistency were good for the personal (α = .80) and social (α = .86) roles subscale scores and composite score (α = .89) for the 8-item Disability, Limitations component of the abbreviated LL-FDI. The estimates of internal consistency were good for the advanced lower body extremity function (α = .88), basic lower body extremity function (α = .86), and upper extremity function (α = .85) subscales and composite score (α = .92) for the 15-item Function component of the abbreviated LL-FDI.

Differences between MS-Types on Components of the Abbreviated LL-FDI

The MANOVA identified a significant main effect of type of MS on subscales of the abbreviated LL-FDI [F (7,281) = 6.20, $p < .001$]. Examination of univariate follow-up analyses indicated that the overall multivariate effect could be best explained by differences in the basic and advanced lower extremity subscales of the Function component of the LL-FDI and personal and social roles subscales of the Disability, Limitations component of the abbreviated LL-FDI (values of $p < .05$). Individuals with RRMS reported fewer limitations with personal and social tasks and less difficulty with advanced and basic lower extremity tasks than did individuals with PPMS and SPMS, and the differences were generally moderate-to-large in magnitude. The mean scores, standard deviations, and effect sizes are provided in table 3.

Table 3. Mean scores on abbreviated LL-FDI subscales by type of multiple sclerosis

	RRMS	PPMS/SPMS	
	M (*SD*)	*M* (*SD*)	*d*
Disability, Frequency Social	13.0 (2.9)	13.5 (2.7)	0.18
Disability, Frequency Personal	17.7 (2.4)	17.3 (2.5)	0.16
Disability, Limitation Social	16.0 (3.5)	14.6 (3.7)	0.39
Disability, Limitation Personal	17.0 (2.9)	15.9 (3.3)	0.36
Function, Advanced Lower Extremity	14.8 (5.6)	10.0 (3.9)	0.86
Function, Basic Lower Extremity	21.6 (3.7)	19.2 (3.9)	0.63
Function, Upper Extremity	19.9 (4.4)	19.2 (3.9)	0.17

Note. RRMS = relapsing-remitting multiple sclerosis. PPMS = primary-progressive multiple sclerosis. SPMS = secondary-progressive multiple sclerosis. M = mean score. SD = standard deviation. d = effect size expressed as Cohen's d.

Correlations between Abbreviated Components of the LL-FDI and Measures of Physical Activity, Walking Mobility, and Neurological Impairment

All correlations between scores from the abbreviated version of the LL-FDI with scores from the measures of physical activity, walking mobility, and neurological impairment were statistically significant and ranged from small to large in magnitude. The correlations indicated that more physically active individuals with MS reported less difficulty in function, more frequent participation in personal and social role activities, and fewer limitations in performance of social and personal role activities. We further note that individuals with greater walking and neurological impairment reported more difficulty in function, less frequent participation in personal and social role activities, and greater limitations in performance of social and personal role activities. The correlations are provided in table 4.

Table 4. Pearson product-moment correlations between scores from the abbreviated version of the LL-FDI and measure of physical activity

LL-FDI component	Physical Activity	Walking Mobility	Neurological Impairment
Disability, Frequency			
1. Personal Roles	.18	−.28	−.28
2. Social Roles	.12	−.13	−.49
Disability, Limitations			
3. Personal Roles	.30	−.47	−.52
4. Social Roles	.24	−.17	−.52
Function			
5. Upper Extremity Function	.23	−.42	−.53
6. Basic Lower Extremity Function	.36	−.64	−.63
7. Advanced Lower Extremity Function	.53	−.77	−.63

Note. All correlations are statistically significant ($p < .05$) based on a one-tailed test. Physical Activity is measured as average accelerometer counts per day. Walking mobility is based on the Patient Determined Disease Steps scale. Neurological impairment is based on the Symptom Inventory.

DISCUSSION

This study confirmed and extended the psychometric properties of the abbreviated LL-FDI in individuals with MS. We were initially interested in confirming the factor structure of the three components (i.e., Function, Frequency, and Limitation) of the LL-FDI and then examining the reliability and the construct validity of the measure based on differences between individuals with RRMS and PPMS/SPMS and correlations with measures of physical activity, walking mobility, and neurological impairment.

Our analyses provided further support for the structural validity, reliability, and construct validity of scores from the Frequency and Limitation scales of the Disability component of the LL-FDI in individuals with MS. The measurement model with two, correlated factors of social and personal roles provided an excellent fit for the 8-items on both the Frequency and Limitation components of the Disability component of the LL-FDI. Subsequent analyses provided evidence of acceptable internal consistency for the subscales and the overall composite score for both the Frequency and Limitation scales of the Disability component of the LL-FDI. Support for the construct validity was based on examination of the difference between individuals with RRMS and PPMS/SPMS in mean scores on the Frequency and Limitation components of the Disability component of the LL-FDI and inspection of relationships with measures of physical activity, walking mobility, and neurological impairment. Those with RRMS reported fewer limitations with personal and social tasks than those with PPMS and SPMS, and physical inactivity, walking immobility, and neurological impairment were associated with less frequent and more limited participation in personal and social activities. Overall, our findings are consistent with previous research (Motl et al., 2007) and provide further support for the interpretation of scores on the Frequency and Limitation Disability components of the LL-FDI as measures of personal and social aspects of disability in those with MS.

Beyond the disability component, our analyses provided further support for the structural validity, reliability, and construct validity of scores from the Functional Limitations component of the LL-FDI. The measurement model with three, correlated factors consisting of advanced lower body extremity function, basic lower body extremity function, and upper extremity function provided a good for the 15-item Function component of the abbreviated LL-FDI. The estimates of internal consistency were good for the three subscales and overall composite scores for the 15-item Function component of the abbreviated LL-FDI. Support for the construct validity was based on examination of the difference between individuals with RRMS and PPMS/SPMS in mean scores on the Functional Limitations components of the LL-FDI and inspection of relationships with the measures of physical activity, walking mobility, and neurological impairment. Those with RRMS reported fewer functional limitations with advanced and basic lower extremity function than those with PPMS and SPMS, and physical inactivity, walking immobility, and neurological impairment were associated with greater functional limitations and the strongest correlations were observed with advanced lower extremity function. Overall, our findings provide preliminary support for the interpretation of scores on the Functional Limitations components of the LL-FDI as measures of advanced and basic lower extremity function and upper extremity function in those with MS.

The abbreviated LL-FDI might represent a major methodological advancement in the study of function and disability in MS. This is based on satisfaction of important considerations when selecting a measure of function and disability in MS, namely sound evidence of psychometric properties and clinical usefulness (Coulthard-Morris, 2000). Our study provided additional evidence for psychometric soundness based on the structural validity, reliability, and construct validity of scores from the abbreviated LL-FDI in a new sample of individuals with MS. Based on the perspective of clinical usefulness, the abbreviated LL-FDI has low time of administration (5-10 minutes) and degree of respondent burden and high degrees of relative ease of use and user-friendliness combined with the provision of a user manual and training guidelines for the original LL-FDI that are equally applicable for the abbreviated LL-FDI. Other strong features of the abbreviated LL-FDI include the conceptual reasoning behind its development and its basis in Nagi's (1976) disablement framework.

Despite our positive preliminary support, there are directions for future research in evaluating the psychometric properties of the abbreviated LL-FDI in individuals with MS. One important direction for future research involves an examination of the sensitivity of the abbreviated LL-FDI based on serial administrations over time in the presence and absence of a treatment for MS, comparisons of the instrument with other criteria of change such as patient or clinician perception, and comparison of the relative responsiveness of the instrument with other instruments of the same entity. Such inquires will provide a clearer picture of the validity of the abbreviated LL-FDI as a measure of function and disability in those with MS.

The continued study of function and disability in MS is important because this is one of the most common neurological diseases among adults 20-50 years of age, affecting approximately 400,000 Americans during the prime years of productivity (NMSS, 2005). Indeed, an estimated 50–80% of individuals with MS are unemployed and disabled within 10 years of disease onset (Rao et al., 1991). The rates of MS and associated unemployment and disability have underscored the importance of examining strategies for reducing functional limitations and disability in this population. Accordingly, future research might consider examining the influence of physical activity on functional limitations and disability in individuals with MS and this could be best accomplished based on Nagi's disablement process model (1976) and the abbreviated LL-FDI. The disablement model and its operational definitions (Verbrugge and Jette, 1994) describe the transitions from pathology (i.e., disease, for example, MS) into impairment (i.e., dysfunction and structural abnormalities in specific body systems, for example, demyelenation of axons in central nervous system), impairment into functional limitations (i.e., restrictions in basic physical and mental actions, for example, walking one mile), and functional limitations into disability (i.e., difficulty doing activities of daily living, for example, activities that are required for one's employment, personal care, and recreation). The disablement model has recently been extended (Stewart, 2003) such that symptoms serve as a step between impairment and functional limitations. Using the abbreviated LL-FDI and a measure of MS-related symptoms, the disablement process model would afford a test of the influence of physical activity on disability, including the possibilities that symptoms and functional limitations serve as entry points for explaining any effect of physical activity on disability in persons with MS.

References

Bentler, P.M. (1990). Comparative fit indexes in structural models. *Psychological Bulletin, 107,* 238–246.

Bollen, K.A. (1989). *Structural Equations with Latent Variables*. New York: Wiley-Interscience.

Coulthard-Morris, L. (2000). Clinical and rehabilitation outcome measures. In J.S. Burks and K.P. Johnson (Eds.), *Multiple sclerosis: Diagnosis, medical management, and rehabilitation* (pp. 221-290). New York, NY: Demos.

Craig, C.L., Marshall, A.L., Sjostrom, M., Bauman, A.E., Booth, M.L., Ainsworth, B. E., et al. (2003). International physical activity questionnaire: 12-country reliability and validity. *Medicine and Science in Sports and Exercis*e, 35, 1381-1395.

Frohman, E.M., Racke, M., and van den Noort, S. (2000). To treat, or not to treat: The therapeutic dilemma of idiopathic monosymptomatic demyelinating syndromes. *Archives of Neurology, 57*, 930-932.

Gosney, J.L., Scott, J.A., Snook, E.M., and Motl, R.W. (2007). Physical activity and multiple sclerosis: Validity of self-report and objective measures. *Family and Community Health, 30,* 144-150.

Guralnik, J.M., and Ferrucci, L. (2003). Assessing the building blocks of function: Utilizing measures of functional limitation. *American Journal of Preventive Medicine, 25*, (Suppl.), 112-121.

Hadjimichael, O., Kerns, R. B., Rizzo, M. A., Cutter, G., and Vollmer, T. (2007). Persistent pain and uncomfortable sensations in persons with multiple sclerosis. *Pain, 127*, 35-41.

Hu, L., and Bentler, P.M. (1999). Cutoff criteria for fit indices in covariance structure analysis: Conventional versus new alternatives. *Structural Equation Modeling, 6,* 1-55.

Jette, A.M., Haley, S.M., Coster, W.J., Kooyoomjian, J.T., Levenson, S., Heeren, T., et al. (2002). Late life function and disability instrument: I. Development and evaluation of the disability component. *Journals of Gerontology A: Biological Sciences and Medical Sciences, 57,* M209-M216.

Lublin, F.D. (2005). Clinical features and diagnosis of multiple sclerosis. *Neurology Clinics, 23,* 1-15.

Marrie, R.A., and Goldman, M. (in press) Validity of performance scales for disability assessment in multiple sclerosis. *Multiple Sclerosis.*

McAuley, E., Konopack, J.F., Motl, R.W., Rosengren, K., and Morris K.S. (2005). Measuring disability and function in older women: Psychometric properties of the late-life function and disability instrument. *Journals of Gerontology A: Biological Sciences and Medical Sciences. 60,* 901-909.

Motl, R.W., McAuley, E., Snook, E. M., and Scott, J. A. (2005). Validity of physical activity measures in ambulatory individuals with multiple sclerosis. *Disability and Rehabilitation, 28,* 1151-1156.

Motl, R.W., Snook, E., Gosney, J. L., and McAuley, E. (2007). Measuring disability and function in individuals with multiple sclerosis: Psychometric properties of the Late-Life Function and Disability Instrument. In P. M. Goldfarb (Ed.), *Psychological tests and testing* (pp. 251-263). Hauppauge, NY: Nova Science Publishers.

Nagi, S.Z. (1976). An epidemiology of disability among adults in the United States. *Milbank Quarterly, 54,* 439-467.

National Multiple Sclerosis Society (2005). *Multiple sclerosis information sourcebook.* New York: Information Resource Center and Library of the National Multiple Sclerosis Society.

Rao, S. M., Leo, G. J., Ellington, L., Nauretz, T., Bernardin, L., and Unverzagt, F. (1991). Cognitive dysfunction in multiple sclerosis: II. Impact on employment and social functioning. *Neurology, 41,* 692-696.

Rudick, R., Antel, J., Confavreux, C., Cutter, G., Ellison, G., Fischer, J., et al. (1996). Clinical outcomes and assessment in multiple sclerosis. *Annals of Neurology, 49,* 169-179.

Runmarker, B., and Andersen, O. (1993). Prognostic factors in multiple sclerosis incident cohort with twenty-five years of follow-up. *Brain, 116,* 117-134.

Schwartz, C.E., Vollmer, T., and Lee, H. (1999) Reliability and validity of two self-report measures of impairment and disability for MS. *Neurology, 52,* 63-70.

Stewart, A.L. (2003). Conceptual challenges in linking physical activity and disability research. *American Journal of Preventive Medicine, 25,* (Suppl.), 137-140.

Verbrugge, L.M., and Jette, A.M. (1994). The disablement process. *Social Science in Medicine, 38,* 1-14.

Weinshenker, B.G., Bass, B., Rice, G.P., Noseworthy, J., Carriere W., Baskerville, J., et al. (1989). The natural history of multiple sclerosis: A geographically based study. Clinical course and disability. *Brain, 112,* 133-146.

In: Multiple Sclerosis Research Progress
Editors: H. Schwarz, L. Walter ISBN: 978-1-60456-570-6
© 2008 Nova Science Publishers, Inc.

Chapter 4

EVALUATION OF STATINS FOR MULTIPLE SCLEROSIS: OPPORTUNITIES AND OBSTACLES

Oliver Neuhaus[1]
Department of Neurology, Kliniken Landkreis Sigmaringen GmbH,
Sigmaringen, Germany

ABSTRACT

Disease-modifying agents currently used in treatment of multiple sclerosis (MS) are only incompletely effective and are often associated with adverse events and high cost. Thus, alternative treatment options are highly desirable. Statins that are inhibitors of 3-hydroxy-3-methylglutaryl coenzyme A (HMG-CoA) reductase are widely prescribed as cholesterol-lowering agents. They may be a future treatment option for MS – either in an add-on therapy regime or alone – as they have been shown to exhibit potent immunomodulatory effects. Several recent reports have demonstrated that statins prevent and reverse chronic and relapsing experimental autoimmune encephalomyelitis (EAE), an animal model of MS. Furthermore, *in vitro* experiments with human immune cells have exhibited an immunomodulatory mode of action of statins comparable to that of interferon-β. An open label clinical trial assessing simvastatin in MS revealed a significant decrease in the number and volume of new MRI lesions and a favourable safety profile. A large multicenter, placebo-controlled phase II clinical trial assessing atorvastatin in patients with clinically isolated syndrome (CIS; a disease that predisposes to development MS) is currently underway. However, prospective placebo-controlled trials of statins in definite MS are difficult to perform due to ethical and financial objections. Furthermore, overly optimistic reports in the popular media as well as often uncontrolled access of MS patients to statins complicate the evaluation of statins as a realistic treatment option for the future. This chapter reviews the current state of HMG-

[1] Department of Neurology, Kliniken Landkreis Sigmaringen GmbH, Hohenzollernstr. 40, D-72488 Sigmaringen Tel.: +49-7571-100-2483. Fax: +49-7571-100-2836. E-Mail: o.neuhaus@klksig.de

CoA reductase inhibitors in the context of their putative mechanisms of action and outlines the next steps necessary to increase the level of evidence concerning their therapeutic use in MS.

Keywords: multiple sclerosis, pathogenesis, immunomodulation, statins

INTRODUCTION

Multiple sclerosis

Multiple sclerosis (MS) is the most common chronic central nervous system (CNS) disorder of the younger adulthood and a major cause of lasting neurological disability in this age group[1]. MS affects more than 1.5 million patients worldwide and is associated with enormous direct and indirect socioeconomic costs.

Pathogenesis

The pathogenesis of MS is still not fully understood, but recent observations shed light on a broad pathogenetic cascade[2,3]. Deviations of immune responses contribute to the formation and perturbation of the MS lesion[4]. The initial inflammatory phase is characterized by selective demyelination, and eventually is paralleled by a neurodegenerative phase with axonal loss and gliosis[2,5]. With ever novel scientific information emerging, concepts regarding the pathogenesis of MS are in constant flux as shown in Figure 1[6]. In genetically susceptible individuals, activation of CNS antigen-specific, encephalitogenic T cells occurs in response to a yet unidentified trigger probably in secondary lymphoid organs. Once activated, these T lymphocytes are able to migrate through the blood-brain barrier and invade the CNS. Reactivated there by intrinsic CNS antigen-presenting cells (APC) including microglia, they release pro-inflammatory cytokines and orchestrate destruction of the myelin sheath by various mechanisms.

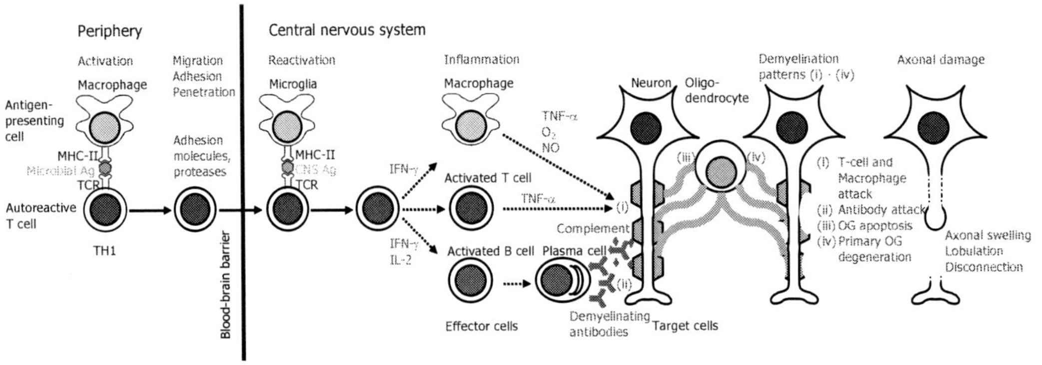

Figure 1. Hypothetical pathogenesis of multiple sclerosis

Via their T-cell receptor (TCR), pro-inflammatory T cells are activated in the periphery by foreign or self antigens (Ag) presented on major histocompatibility complex class II (MHC-II) by antigen-presenting cells (APC), including dendritic cells and B cells. Activated T cells migrate to, adhere at and penetrate through the blood-brain barrier, a step mediated by adhesion molecules, proteases and chemokines. Inside the central nervous system (CNS), T cells are reactivated in the context of MHC-II on resident APC, predominantly microglia cells. These reactivated T cells secrete pro-inflammatory cytokines, such as interferon (IFN)-γ or interleukin (IL)-2 and induce CNS inflammation by subsequent activation of macrophages, other T cells and B cells as effector cells. Macrophages and T cells attack the oligodendrocytic myelin sheath by cytotoxic mediators, mainly tumor necrosis factor (TNF)-α, oxygen (O_2) radicals and nitric oxide (NO). B cells differentiate to plasma cells that secrete demyelinating antibodies. They can guide and activate macrophages or ignite the complement cascade with assembly of the membrane attack complex which causes pore formation in myelin membranes. Modified from Ref. 6, with permission from Elsevier.

Pathologically, four different patterns of demyelination have been observed, namely

(i) T-cell and macrophage-mediated demyelination,
(ii) antibody-mediated demyelination involving complement activation,
(iii) distal oligodendrogliopathy, and oligodendrocyte apoptosis,
(iv) primary oligodendrocyte degeneration[4].

Interestingly, the presence of pattern (iii), oligodendrocyte apoptosis, has recently been demonstrated even in very early MS lesions, suggesting that at least in some patients a degenerative process may be an early event in this disorder[7]. In addition, recent evidence suggests that axonal loss responsible for irreversible disability occurs already early in the disease course and – as the disease evolves – predominates the histopathological features[2, 8].

Current treatment options

Until the early 1990s, corticosteroids were the sole available therapy. However, the activity of these agents was limited to shortening acute MS attacks. In addition, a number of immunosuppressive agents (i.e.,inhibitors of crucial components of the immune system causing generalized immune dysfunction) were used off label, e.g., azathioprine (licensed for treatment of MS in several countries), methotrexate or cyclophosphamide[9]. The potential beneficial effects of these therapies in MS were limited by systemic adverse effects, such as increased risk of neoplasia or infection.

More recently, two classes of immunomodulatory agents have been approved for the treatment of relapsing-remitting MS, namely interferon-β (IFN-β1a and IFN-β1b) and glatiramer acetate (GA)[10-14]. Immunomodulators - without generally suppressing immunological properties - shift immune responses from pro-inflammatory autoimmune conditions (mediated by T-helper (TH)-1 cytokines released from autoreactive T cells) towards a more beneficial anti-inflammatory environment (mediated through TH2 cytokines secreted by regulatory T cells).

Mitoxantrone, a chemotherapeutic agent, has been approved for active forms of relapsing-remitting and secondary progressive MS[15,16].

More recently, natalizumab, a monoclonal antibody against α4-integrin (an adhesion molecule expressed on T lymphocytes) targeting T-cell migration exhibited excellent effects on relapse rate and magnetic resonance imaging (MRI) parameters in clinical trials[17] and thus has been approved for treatment of RRMS[18].

For current therapeutic strategies and future treatment options in MS see Refs.[6,19]. All currently approved pharmacotherapies for MS, both immunomodulatory and immunosuppressive, exhibit only limited efficacy and all agents have to be administered parenterally. Patients not infrequently suffer from potentially serious adverse events. In addition, all disease-modifying drugs approved for the treatment of MS are exceptionally expensive. Thus, alternative treatment options are warranted that provide good efficacy, oral application, negligible side effects and low cost[20].

HMG-CoA reductase inhibitors

Hints have emerged that one group of substances may fulfil most of the criteria mentioned above. Statins, which are widely used as lipid-lowering agents,

i. have been demonstrated to exhibit immunomodulatory effects *in vitro* and in animal models of MS
ii. are administered orally
iii. have a well-established favourable safety profile
iv. cost about 10% of the currently available disease-modifying drugs against MS

Statins (Figure 2) are inhibitors of the 3-hydroxy-3-methylglutaryl coenzyme A (HMG-CoA) reductase, an enzyme that catalyzes the rate-limiting step of the cholesterol biosynthesis pathway.

Statins have been in clinical use for almost two decades and are among the most frequently sold medications. In fact, atorvastatin is believed to be the current world's biggest single hot seller with annual sales of approximately US-$10 billion.

Safety considerations

The overall safety profile of statins is favourable[21]. Rare – though unpredictable – side effects include hepatotoxicity (< 3%) and myopathy (< 0.5%) with a very low risk (< 0.1%) of severe rhabdomyolysis[22]. The risk of rhabdomyolysis threatening kidney function by myoglobinuria is not trivial and obviously dependent on the statin and concomitant medication (especially fibrates and niacin) used[23,24]. Cerivastatin, an HMG-CoA reductase inhibitor potently lowering cholesterol, induced lethal rhabdomyolysis in some 50 patients leading to its withdrawal from the market[25]. In order to avoid statin-associated adverse events, patient's liver and muscle enzymes should be monitored carefully and patients have to be made aware of early signs of hepatopathy and myopathy.

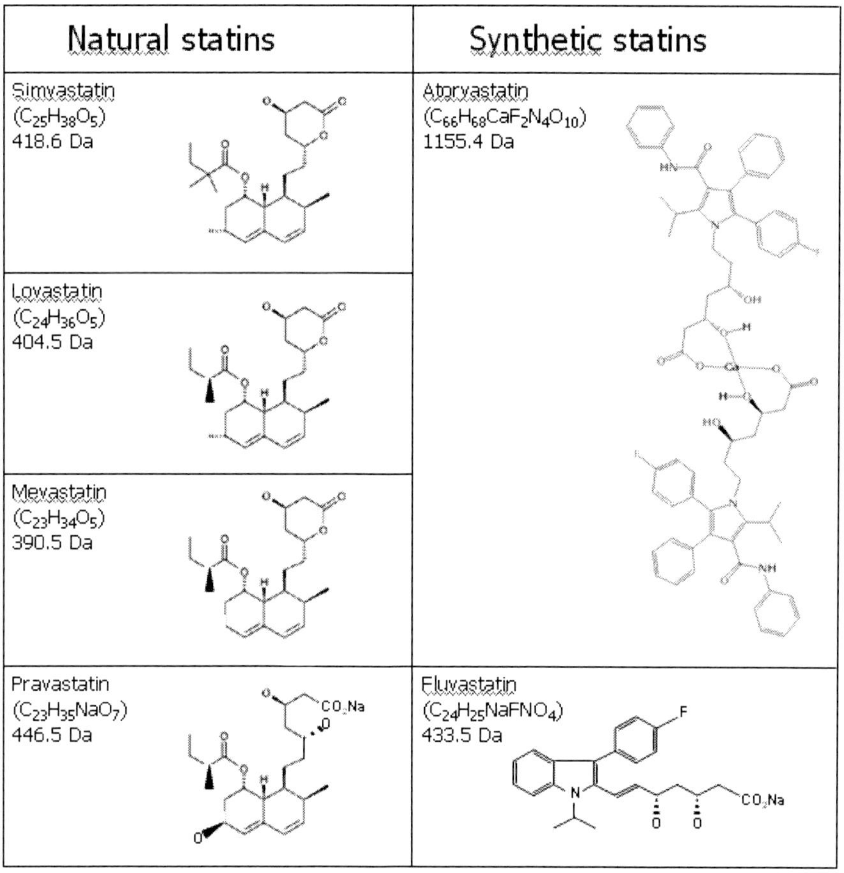

Figure 2. Structural features of important statins
Simvastatin, lovastatin, mevastatin and pravastatin are natural (fungus-derived) statins; atorvastatin and fluvastatin are synthetic.

Effects of statins beyond cholesterol lowering

Recently, it was demonstrated that statins exhibit effects far beyond pure cholesterol lowering[26]. They decrease cardiovascular-related morbidity and mortality[27]. Antineoplastic effects have been reported[28,29]. They even may be beneficial in Alzheimer's disease[30] or in stroke (although the blood cholesterol levels as a risk factor in ischemic stroke has yet to be clearly established)[31]. Also, statins have been recognized as immunomodulators for many years[32-37]. In a recently published double-blind, placebo-controlled trial of atorvastatin in rheumatoid arthritis, modest but significant beneficial effects of the HMG-CoA reductase inhibitor were observed[38].

Statins in experimental autoimmune encephalomyelitis

Recently, a series of publications brought statins into the focus of interest as a potential therapy for MS[39-43]. Statins have been shown to ameliorate or even prevent disease expression in experimental autoimmune encephalomyelitis (EAE), an animal model of MS. Immunologically, a shift from pro-inflammatory towards anti-inflammatory conditions was consistently observed, confirming the immunomodulatory potential of statins.

Statins in vitro

In vitro studies on human peripheral blood lymphocytes revealed that simvastatin, lovastatin and mevastatin exhibited strong anti-inflammatory properties comparable to those of IFN-β1b[44]. Interestingly, the combination of statins and interferon IFN-β1b exhibited additive anti-inflammatory effects. However, partial pro-inflammatory effects induced by statins by heightened secretion of IFN-γ and interleukin (IL)-12 were also observed[44]. This latter observation has recently been confirmed in the mouse system, as simvastatin has been demonstrated to enhance lipopolysaccharaide (LPS)-induced IL-12p40 production by murine macrophages[45].

Putative mechanisms of action of statins in multiple sclerosis

Several mechanisms of action by which statins regulate the immune system have been described.

By inhibition of the product of HMG-CoA reductase, mevalonate, the synthesis of other important intermediates of the cholesterol biosynthetic pathway is also impaired, likely explaining the multimodal effects of statins. Farnesylpyrophosphate (F-PP) and geranylgeranylpyrophosphate (GG-PP) are important lipid attachments used in the posttranslational modification of several proteins including the small guanosine triphosphate (GTP)-binding proteins Ras, Rac and Rho[46]. Only the attachment of F-PP or GG-PP, termed isoprenylation, permits subsequent activation and membrane translocation of these proteins, which is crucial for a variety of cellular functions, such as cell shape, motility, secretion, differentiation and proliferation. Thus, prevention of isoprenylation of Rho by statins induces the accumulation of inactive Rho molecules in the cytosol and inhibits cellular functions vital for the activation of various cell types, including that of encephalitogenic leukocytes (Figure 3)[37,47].

An alternatively suggested effector pathway of statins is via cholesterol itself[48]. Cellular membranes contain microdomains with relatively high cholesterol concentrations – so-called lipid rafts. These rafts bear important immunological molecules, e.g., Fc receptors, and are essential for vital immune functions[49]. Statins are able to disintegrate the lipid rafts affecting those cellular functions (Figure 3).

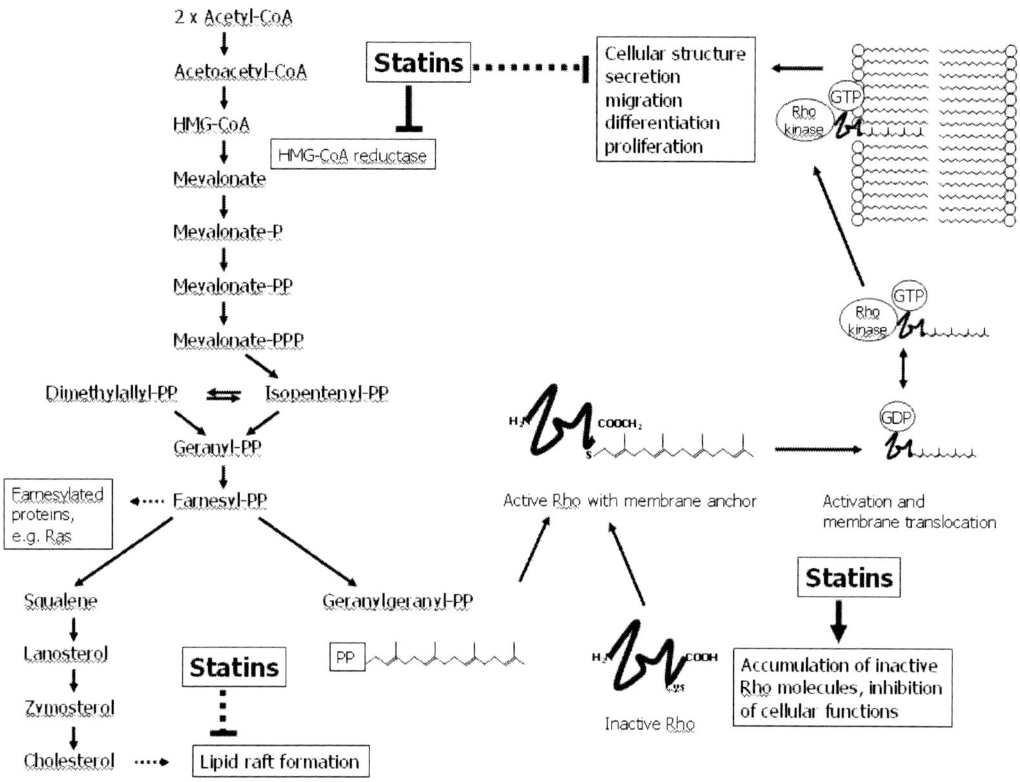

Figure 3. Cholesterol biosynthesis and isoprenylation of Rho.

Farnesylpyrophosphate (-PP) and its derivative, geranylgeranyl-PP are lipid attachments for the posttranslational modification of immunologically important proteins (e.g., Ras, Rac, Rho). This "isoprenylation" permits subsequent activation and membrane translocation of this type of proteins that is crucial for a variety of cellular functions. Isoprenylated Rho binds to GDP and acts as molecular switch between a dormant GDP-binding and an active GTP-binding state that exerts its biological function by binding to Rho kinase. Prevention of isoprenylation of Rho by statins induces the accumulation of inactive Rho molecules in the cytosol and inhibits cellular functions vital for leukocyte activation. Alternatively, statins act by disrupting the integrity of lipid rafts containing important immunological molecules. All HMG-CoA reductase dependent effects of statins can be antagonized by L-mevalonate. HMG-CoA = 3-hydroxy-3-methylglutaryl coenzyme A; P = phosphate residue; GDP = guanosinediphosphate; GTP = guanosinetriphosphate. Modified from Ref. 37, with permission from Elsevier.

Nearly all immunomodulatory effects of statins, including both those mediated by inhibition of isoprenylation of small GTP-binding proteins and those by disruption of lipid raft integrity, can be reversed by treatment with L-mevalonate, the product of HMG-CoA reductase, indicating that statin-induced immunomodulation is mediated through inhibition of the mevanolate pathway. However, there is at least one exception. Statins have been observed to directly inhibit leukocyte function antigen (LFA)-1[50], a cellular adhesion molecule that has key roles in both T-cell activation and migration into the brain[51].

A number of immunological effects of statins have been described thus far. For example, statins block IFN-γ-inducible transcription of the major histocompatibility complex (MHC) class II transactivator (CIITA), which regulates nearly all MHC class II gene expression and consequently inhibits activation of $CD4^+$ T lymphocytes[40,52]. Furthermore, in animal models a TH2 shift was consistently demonstrated[40,41], whereas *in vitro* experiments revealed that statins heightened secretion of both TH2 and some TH1 cytokines[44,45]. An overview of current knowledge on the mechanisms of action of statins in MS is given in the table.

Table. Immune mechanisms of statins

Immune mechanism	Reference
↓ Expression and secretion of pro-inflammatory cytokines	40,43,57
Cytokine shift from T-helper 1 to T-helper 2	40,43
↓ MHC class II expression	40,44,52
↓ Proliferation of macrophages	58,59
↓ Expression of adhesion molecules	44,50,60,61
↓ Expression and secretion of matrix metalloproteinases	44,59
↓ Secretion of chemokines	62
↓ Expression of chemokine receptors	44
↓ Activation of B lymphocytes	63
↓ T-cell proliferation	34,40-42,44
↓ Lymphocyte migration	42
Mediation of neuroprotection	61,64

↓, Inhibitory effect.

Possible action sites of statins in the immunopathogenesis of MS are shown in Figure 4.

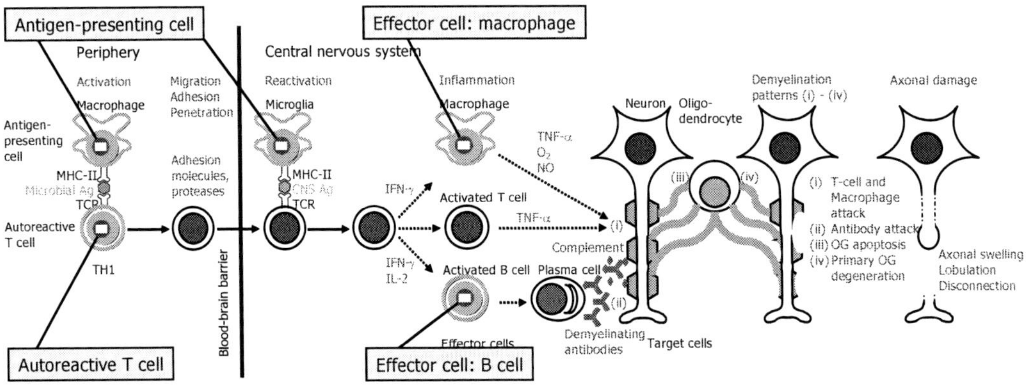

Figure 4. Action sites of statins in the pathogenesis of multiple sclerosis
Statins have been shown to exert a variety of inhibitory effects on autoreactive T cells, B cells, macrophages and other antigen-presenting cells. See Figure 1.

Statins in multiple sclerosis – clinical data

Two smaller studies examining treatment effects of statins on patients with MS have been presented recently. Sena et al., reported a small open-label study with lovastatin in MS[53].

Seven patients with relapsing-remitting MS and at least two relapses during the previous two years received 20 mg lovastatin for twelve months. There were no serious adverse events. Although no clinical changes were observed, magnetic resonance imaging (MRI) revealed partial treatment effects in this small cohort. Vollmer et al. published the results of an open-label phase II study with simvastatin in MS[54]. Twenty-eight patients with relapsing-remitting MS with active disease on MRI scans were treated for six months with 80 mg of simvastatin daily. Serial MRI scans were obtained at months 4, 5 and 6 during treatment. A 44% reduction in the mean number of new gadolinium-enhancing lesions ($p<0.0001$) and a 41% reduction in the mean volume of new gadolinium-enhancing lesions ($p=0.0018$) were observed. No serious adverse events and no clinical changes were noted in this short study.

Patients enrolled in the latter trial were screened for high pre-treatment MRI activity, and because in both the Sena and the Vollmer trial there were no placebo arms, the possibility remains that the positive results could be based on regression to the mean.

Statins in multiple sclerosis – future directions

Based on EAE and in vitro data and on two small open-label clinical studies, the level of evidence that statins have a treatment effect does not exceed class IV and thus is still low. For further evaluation of the role of HMG-CoA reductase inhibitors in MS prospective, randomized, placebo-controlled, blinded trials are highly warranted. Statins should be assessed both alone and in combination with approved MS treatments. Those trials should answer the question if statins – either alone or combined with an established disease modifying drug – represent a viable therapeutic option in MS.

A multicenter randomized, placebo-controlled trial that anticipates enrolling 152 patients has recently started. This phase II trial will evaluate whether treatment with high-dose atorvastatin (80 mg daily) in patients that have experienced their first demyelinating attack (a clinically isolated syndrome, CIS) will decrease the risk of developing MS activity.

Evaluation of statins in multiple sclerosis – obstacles

The results of the prospective controlled trial of atorvastatin in CIS will be most helpful. This trial – if establishing atorvastatin effective – may lead to its approval for the treatment of CIS. However, for the assessment of HMG-CoA reductase inhibitors as a treatment option in MS itself or even for their approval, health authorities most probably demand class I evidence obtained from controlled clinical trials in MS. Although efforts by several groups are currently being made to plan and organize such trials, several obstacles have emerged.

Methodological problems of study design

It is matter of intense discussion which clinical or paraclinical parameter could reflect significant advantages of new agents against current drugs, especially if assessed in add-on trials. Measurement of relapse rate and/or sustained progression as primary outcome measures requires long-term trials with large patient numbers. MRI parameters are more promising but still insufficient for health authorities.

Ethical problems

As several drugs are approved for treatment of MS, placebo-controlled trials in MS are ethically possible only under stringent restrictions. In this regard, it is considered unethical to treat individuals for 24 months or longer with placebo only. Thus, cross-over studies would be more feasible, but the probability of reaching a clinical primary endpoint decreases. Moreover, true placebo groups become increasingly difficult to recruit as self-medication with statins cannot be ruled out. A possible solution would be a "virtual" placebo group created through merging placebo data from previous clinical trials[55]. The use of such an experimental approach has yet to be validated.

Financial obstacles

Clinical trials with large patient numbers, long duration and serial MRI scans are extremely expensive and easily reach cost exceeding several million US-$. There are several reasons why incentives to conduct clinical statin trials may be lacking for pharmaceutical companies. Many statins that have been evaluated in animal models or *in vitro* have lost or will loose their patent protection in the near future. In addition, comparing possible sales market of statins in MS to the existing sales market of statins in cardiovascular diseases, MS must be denoted "orphan disease". Furthermore, producers of generic statins are generally not interested in supporting clinical trials, governmental research funding institutions rarely support drug research, and health insurance companies that would profit the most from approval of statins for treatment of MS do not possess the required research budget. Manufacturers of currently approved disease-modifying drugs against MS may be interested in add-on trials but simultaneously they may fear the results of these trials because of their shareholder value.

Statins in the media

Although the level of evidence is far too limited for recommendation of statins for the treatment of MS, enthusiastic reports regarding the potential efficacy of statins in MS have been released in the popular media. It is our personal experience that some fellow physicians already provide off-label use of statins, either as add-on therapy, or as replacement of approved therapies. Since July 2004, patients in the UK have been able to receive simvastatin without a prescription as an "over the counter medication". Overly optimistic portrayal of potential statin-efficacy in MS may lead to self-medication with these agents.

What are the next steps?

In order to circumvent the scenario mentioned above, at least four multinational multicenter randomized placebo-controlled trials may be organized:

(i) statin plus IFN-β vs. placebo plus IFN-β;
(ii) statin plus GA vs. placebo plus GA;
(iii) statin plus mitoxantrone vs. placebo plus mitoxantrone;
(iv) statin alone vs. placebo alone.

Private companies, governmental research funding institutions, health insurances, and private money givers may need to participate together in order to bear the costs of such a large effort. Only then the level of evidence concerning the role of HMG-CoA reductase inhibitors in MS can be obtained.

As both the approved disease-modifying agents and statins share common mechanisms of action in the inflammatory cascade of MS, yet differ in others, combinations of these agents are reasonable. Consistent with this notion, *in vitro* experiments exhibited additive effects of IFN-β1b and statins[44]. In EAE, the combination of suboptimal doses of GA and atorvastatin ameliorated the clinical course of the disease which was not observed with the GA or atorvastatin alone[56].

CONCLUSION

In recent years there have been major advances in understanding how cellular and humoral immune responses contribute to the pathogenesis of MS. If today's obstacles of clinical research and trial design could be overcome and if statins were proven effective, they could offer a potential alternative to currently available drugs.

REFERENCES

[1] Noseworthy, J.H., Lucchinetti, C., Rodriguez, M. et al. (2000). Medical progress: multiple sclerosis. *N Engl J Med,* 343, 938-52.

[2] Hemmer, B., Archelos, J.J., Hartung, H.P. (2002). New concepts in the immunopathogenesis of multiple sclerosis. *Nat Rev Neurosci,* 3, 291-301.

[3] Zamvil, S.S., Steinman, L. (2003). Diverse targets for intervention during inflammatory and neurodegenerative phases of multiple sclerosis. *Neuron,* 38, 685-8.

[4] Lassmann, H., Brück, W., Lucchinetti, C. (2001). Heterogeneity of multiple sclerosis pathogenesis: implications for diagnosis and therapy. *Trends Mol Med,* 7, 115-21.

[5] Steinman L. (2001). Multiple sclerosis: a two-stage disease. *Nat Immunol,* 2, 762-4.

[6] Neuhaus, O., Archelos, J.J., Hartung, H.P. (2003). Immunomodulation in multiple sclerosis: from immunosuppression to neuroprotection. *Trends Pharmacol Sci,* 24, 131-8.

[7] Barnett, M.H., Prineas, J.W. (2004). Relapsing and remitting multiple sclerosis: pathology of the newly forming lesion. *Ann Neurol,* 55, 458-68.
[8] Trapp, B.D., Ransohoff, R.M., Rudick, R. (1999). Axonal pathology in multiple sclerosis: relationship to neurologic disability. *Curr Opin Neurol,* 12, 295-302.
[9] Fernandez, O., Fernandez, V., De Ramon, E. (2004). Azathioprine and methotrexate in multiple sclerosis. *J Neurol Sci,* 223, 29-34.
[10] The IFNB Multiple Sclerosis Study Group. Interferon beta-1b is effective in relapsing-remitting multiple sclerosis: I. Clinical results of a multicenter, randomized, double-blind, placebo-controlled trial. *Neurology, (*1993). 43, 655-61.
[11] Jacobs, L.D., Cookfair, D.L., Rudick, R.A. et al. (1996). Intramuscular interferon beta-1a for disease progression in exacerbating-remitting multiple sclerosis. The Multiple Sclerosis Collaborative Research Group (MSCRG). *Ann Neurol,* 39, 285-94.
[12] PRISMS (Prevention of Relapses and Disability by Interferon beta-1a Subcutaneously in Multiple Sclerosis) Study Group. Randomised double-blind placebo-controlled study of interferon beta-1a in relapsing/remitting multiple sclerosis. *Lancet, (*1998). 352, 1498-504.
[13] Johnson, K.P., Brooks, B.R., Cohen, J.A. et al. (1995). Copolymer 1 reduces relapse rate and improves disability in relapsing-remitting multiple sclerosis: results of a phase III multicenter, double-blind, placebo-controlled trial. The Copolymer 1 Multiple Sclerosis Study Group. *Neurology,* 45, 1268-76.
[14] Kieseier, B.C., Hartung, H.P. (2003). Current disease-modifying therapies in multiple sclerosis. *Semin Neurol,* 23, 133-45.
[15] Hartung, H.P., Gonsette, R., König, N. et al. (2002). A placebo-controlled, double-blind, randomised, multicentre trial of mitoxantrone in progressive multiple sclerosis. *Lancet,* 360, 2018-25.
[16] Neuhaus, O., Kieseier, B.C., Hartung, H.P. (2004). Mitoxantrone (Novantrone) in multiple sclerosis - new insights. *Exp Rev Neurotherapeutics,* 4, 17-26.
[17] Miller, D.H., Khan, O.A., Sheremata, W.A. et al. (2003). A controlled trial of natalizumab for relapsing multiple sclerosis. *N Engl J Med,* 348, 15-23.
[18] Rice, G.P., Hartung, H.P., Calabresi, P.A. (2005). Anti-alpha4 integrin therapy for multiple sclerosis. Mechanisms and rationale. *Neurology,* Apr 7 (Epub ahead of print).
[19] Wiendl, H., Kieseier, B.C. (2003). Disease-modifying therapies in multiple sclerosis: an update on recent and ongoing trials and future strategies. *Exp Opin Invest Drugs,* 12, 689-712.
[20] Polman, C.H., Uitdehaag, B.M.J. (2003). New and emerging treatment options for multiple sclerosis. *Lancet Neurol,* 2, 563-6.
[21] Davidson, M.H. (2001). Safety profiles for the HMG-CoA reductase inhibitors: treatment and trust. *Drugs,* 61, 197-206.
[22] Gotto, A.M.J. (2003). Safety and statin therapy: reconsidering the risks and benefits. *Arch Intern Med,* 163, 657-9.
[23] Wortmann, R.L. (2002). Lipid-lowering agents and myopathy. *Curr Opin Rheumatol,* 14, 643-7.
[24] Thompson, P.D., Clarkson, P., Karas, R.H. (2003). Statin-associated myopathy. *Jama,* 289, 1681-90.

[25] Staffa, J.A., Chang, J., Green, L.(2002). Cerivastatin and reports of fatal rhabdomyolysis. *N Engl J Med,* 346, 539-40.

[26] Massy, Z.A., Guijarro, C. (2001). Statins: effects beyond cholesterol lowering. *Nephrol Dial Transplant,* 16, 1738-41.

[27] Larosa, J.C., He, J., Vupputuri, S. (1999). Effect of statins on risk of coronary disease: a meta-analysis of randomized controlled trials. *Jama,* 282, 2340-6.

[28] Chan, K.K.W., Oza, A.M., Siu, L.L. (2003). The statins as anticancer agents. *Clin Cancer Res,* 9, 10-9.

[29] Jakobisiak, M., Golab, J. (2003). Potential antitumor effects of statins. *Int J Oncol,* 23, 1055-69.

[30] Jick, H., Zornberg, G.L., Jick, S.S. et al. (2000). Statins and the risk of dementia. *Lancet,* 356, 1627-31.

[31] White, H.D., Simes, R.J., Anderson, N.E. et al. (2000). Pravastatin therapy and the risk of stroke. *N Engl J Med,* 343, 317-26.

[32] Cutts, J.L., Scallen, T.J., Watson, J. et al. (1989). Role of mevalonic acid in the regulation of natural killer cell cytotoxicity. *J Cell Physiol,* 139, 550-7.

[33] Kobashigawa, J.A., Katznelson, S., Laks, H. et al. (1995). Effects of pravastatin on outcomes after cardiac transplantation. *N Engl J Med,* 333, 621-7.

[34] Kurakata, S., Kada, M., Shimada, Y. et al. (1996). Effects of different inhibitors of 3-hydroxy-3-methylglutaryl coenzyme A (HMG-CoA) reductase, pravastatin sodium and simvastatin, on sterol synthesis and immunological functions in human lymphocytes in vitro. *Immunopharmacology,* 34, 51-61.

[35] Weitz-Schmidt, G. (2002). Statins as anti-inflammatory agents. *Trends Pharmacol Sci,* 23, 482-6.

[36] Baker, D., Adamson, P., Greenwood, J. (2003). Potential of statins for the treatment of multiple sclerosis. *Lancet Neurol,* 2, 9-10.

[37] Neuhaus, O., Stüve, O., Zamvil, S.S. et al. (2004). Are statins a treatment option for multiple sclerosis? *Lancet Neurol,* 3, 369-71.

[38] McCarey, D.W., McInnes, I.B., Madhok, R. et al. (2004). Trial of Atorvastatin in Rheumatoid Arthritis (TARA): double-blind, randomised placebo-controlled trial. *Lancet,* 363, 2015 21.

[39] Stanislaus, R., Pahan, K., Singh, A.K. et al. (1999). Amelioration of experimental allergic encephalomyelitis in Lewis rats by lovastatin. *Neurosci Lett,* 269, 71-4.

[40] Youssef, S., Stüve, O., Patarroyo, J.C. et al. (2002). The HMG-CoA reductase inhibitor, atorvastatin, promotes a Th2 bias and reverses paralysis in central nervous system autoimmune disease. *Nature,* 420, 78-84.

[41] Aktas, O., Waiczies, S., Smorodchenko, A. et al. (2003). Treatment of relapsing paralysis in experimental encephalomyelitis by targeting Th1 cells through atorvastatin. *J Exp Med,* 197, 725-33.

[42] Greenwood, J., Walters, C.E., Pryce, G. et al. (2003). Lovastatin inhibits brain endothelial cell Rho-mediated lymphocyte migration and attenuates experimental autoimmune encephalomyelitis. *Faseb J,* 17, 905-7.

[43] Nath, N., Giri, S., Prasad, R. et al. (2004). Potential targets of 3-hydroxy-3-methylglutaryl coenzyme a reductase inhibitor for multiple sclerosis therapy. *J Immunol,* 172, 1273-86.

[44] Neuhaus, O., Strasser-Fuchs, S., Fazekas, F. et al. (2002). Statins as immunomodulators: comparison with interferon-beta1b in MS. *Neurology,* 59, 990-7.

[45] Matsumoto, M., Einhaus, D., Gold, E.S. et al. (2004). Simvastatin augments lipopolysaccharide-induced proinflammatory responses in macrophages by differential regulation of the c-Fos and c-Jun transcription factors. *J Immunol,* 172, 7377-84.

[46] Takemoto, M., Liao, J.K. (2001). Pleiotropic effects of 3-hydroxy-3-methylglutaryl coenzyme A reductase inhibitors. *Arterioscler Thromb Vasc Biol,* 21, 1712-9.

[47] Singh, R., Wang, B., Shirvaikar, A. et al. (1999). The IL-1 receptor and Rho directly associate to drive cell activation in inflammation. *J Clin Invest,* 103, 1561-70.

[48] Kirsch, C., Eckert, G.P., Mueller, W.E. (2003). Statin effects on cholesterol micro-domains in brain plasma membranes. *Biochem Pharmacol,* 65, 843-56.

[49] Hillyard, D.Z., Jardine, A.G., McDonald, K.J. et al. (2004). Fluvastatin inhibits raft dependent Fc-gamma receptor signalling in human monocytes. *Atherosclerosis,* 172, 219-28.

[50] Weitz-Schmidt, G., Welzenbach, K., Brinkmann, V. et al. (2001). Statins selectively inhibit leukocyte function antigen-1 by binding to a novel regulatory integrin site. *Nat Med,* 7, 687-92.

[51] Archelos, J.J., Hartung, H.P. (1997). The role of adhesion molecules in multiple sclerosis: biology, pathogenesis and therapeutic implications. *Mol Med Today,* 3, 310-21.

[52] Kwak, B., Mulhaupt, F., Myit, S. et al. (2000). Statins as a newly recognized type of immunomodulator. *Nat Med,* 6, 1399-402.

[53] Sena, A., Pedrosa, R., Morais, M.G. (2003). Therapeutic potential of lovastatin in multiple sclerosis. *J Neurol,* 250, 754-5.

[54] Vollmer, T., Key, L., Durkalski, V. et al. (2004). Oral simvastatin treatment in relapsing-remitting multiple sclerosis. *Lancet,* 363, 1607-8.

[55] Daumer, M., Kessner, S., Lederer, C. et al. (2003). Modelling placebo groups for clinical trials. *Mult Scler,* 9 (Supplement 1), S22 (Abstract).

[56] Stüve, O., Youssef, S., Dunn, S. et al. (2004). Atorvastatin enhances the clinically beneficial effects of glatiramer acetate in experimental autoimmune encephalomyelitis through induction of a TH2 phenotype. *Neurology,* 62 (Supplement 5), A438 (Abstract).

[57] Pahan, K., Sheikh, F.G., Namboodiri, A.M. et al. (1997). Lovastatin and phenylacetate inhibit the induction of nitric oxide synthase and cytokines in rat primary astrocytes, microglia, and macrophages. *J Clin Invest,* 100, 2671-9.

[58] Sakai, M., Kobori, S., Matsumura, T. et al. (1997). HMG-CoA reductase inhibitors suppress macrophage growth induced by oxidized low density liproprotein. *Atherosclerosis,* 133, 51-9.

[59] Aikawa, M., Rabkin, E., Sugiyama, S. et al. (2001). An HMG-CoA reductase inhibitor, cerivastatin, suppresses growth of macrophages expressing matrix metalloproteinases, and tissue factor in vivo, and in vitro. *Circulation,* 103, 276-83.

[60] Niwa, S., Totsuka, T., Hayashi, S. (1996). Inhibitory effect of fluvastatin, an HMG-CoA reductase inhibitor, on the expression of adhesion molecules on human monocyte cell line. *Int J Immunopharmacol,* 18, 669-75.

[61] Honjo, M., Tanihara, H., Nishijima, K. et al. (2002). Statin inhibits leukocyte-endothelial interaction and prevents neuronal death induced by ischemia-reperfusion injury in the rat retina. *Arch Ophthalmol,* 120, 1707-13.

[62] Diomede, L., Albani, D., Sottocorno, M. et al. (2001). In vivo anti-inflammatory effects of statins is mediated by nonsterol mevalonate products. *Arterioscler Thromb Vasc Biol,* 21, 1327-32.

[63] Rudich, S.M., Mongini, P.K.A., Perez, R.V.et al. (1998). HMG-CoA reductase inhibitors pravastatin and simvastatin inhibit human B-lymphocyte activation. *Transplant Proc,* 30, 992-5.

[64] Zacco, A., Togo, J., Spence, K. et al. (2003). 3-Hydroxy-3-methylglutaryl coenzyme A reductase inhibitors protect cortical neurons from excitotoxicity. *J Neurosci,* 23, 11104-11.

In: Multiple Sclerosis Research Progress
Editors: H. Schwarz, L. Walter
ISBN: 978-1-60456-570-6
© 2008 Nova Science Publishers, Inc.

Chapter 5

COMPUTERIZED CONTENT ANALYSIS OF SPEECH FOR THE ASSESSMENT OF MENTAL FUNCTION IN MULTIPLE SCLEROSIS PATIENTS

***Stanley van den Noort*[*], *Louis A. Gottschalk*[**] *and Robert J. Bechtel*[***]**

INTRODUCTION

Artificial intelligence software has been developed and validated that is capable of providing computerized content analysis of speech and verbal texts to measure neuropsychiatric states and traits as well as suggesting, at any one time during the course of a medical disorder, possible neuropsychiatric diagnoses derived from the Diagnostic and Statistical Manual (DSM IV) of the American Psychiatric Association (1994)[1]. The application of such a software program during the onset, course, and treatment of multiple sclerosis offers an objective supplement to other measurement procedures applied to this disorder.

The software program, when used as an assessment tool on speech samples from multiple sclerosis or other patients, provides scores on a large number of content analysis scales, compares these scores to already programmed norms for each of these content analysis scales, indicates how many standard deviations these scores differ (if at all) from the expected norms, enabling the clinician to determine the patient's current mental status and its changes over time and with and/or without treatment. The content analysis scales that have been developed and tested for reliability and validity include: Anxiety scale (and six subscales), Hostility Outward Scale (and two subscales), Hostility Inward Scale, Ambivalent Hostility

* Department of Neurology, University of California, Irvine, CA 92697
** Department of Psychiatry, University of California, Irvine, CA 92697
*** Eclectic Computing Concepts, 1650 West Virginia Parkway, Suite 200, McKinney, Texas 75069

Scale, Social Alienation-Personal Disorganization Scale, Cognitive Impairment Scale, Depression Scale (and seven subscales), Health and Health/Sickness Scale, Achievement Strivings Scale, Hope Scale, Human Relations Scale, Dependency Scale, Dependency-Frustration Scale, Quality of Life Scale.

Initially each of these content analysis scales had to be scored by human scorers trained up to an acceptable criterion level[2,3,4]. A computerized capacity to perform the scoring of the application of these content analysis scales was developed by Bechtel[5], Gottschalk[6,7], Gottschalk and Bechtel[8,9].

The patient's recorded speech sample is transcribed into text format in a machine-readable form. The software program PCAD 2000 (Gottschalk and Bechtel, 1999-2003)[10] :

- reads the verbal sample,
- breaks it down into grammatical clauses (which is the smallest unit it is programmed to score),
- identifies the meanings (semantics) conveyed by the clause,
- analyzes which content analysis scale (s) items are relevant to the message,
- tabulates the occurrence of these items and
- assigns predetermined weights to these items separately and where appropriate to each content analysis scale,
- calculates a score for each content analysis scale,
- compares the score obtained to empirically determined norms, and
- reports how many standard deviations (if any) the obtained score differs from the norm for each Scale.

If the scores do not deviate from the norms on any content analysis scales, the program indicates that no psychiatric disorder is suggested using the criteria described in the Diagnostic and Statistical Manual, Fourth Edition of the American Psychiatric Association (American Psychiatric Assn, 1994). On the other hand, if there are significant standard deviations from norms on some content analysis scales, the software program, using only these criteria, suggests a number of possible neuropsychiatric diagnostic classifications that the program user might consider. The norm on each content analysis was obtained from scoring verbal samples from over 100 medically and psychiatrically health adults and children. The computer software program uses Lisp and was written by Dr. Robert Bechtel. The software holds a dictionary of over 300,000 words and includes American idiomatic and slang expressions, and it associates these with certain neuropsychobiological states categorized in the items underlying each content analysis scale. The dictionary can be enlarged at will to understand the meaning of any expressions or jargon specific to any environment. These associations, along with ordinary grammatical rules, permit strings of words to be parsed into grammaticaal clauses. The clauses are then content analyzed, and the result is reviewed by a computer-generated list of scoreable candidates. Once the list is compiled, each scoreable candidate clause is examined by a set of scale-dependent procedures that assess the structure, and more importantly the score marking and weighting, to determine the validity of the scoring for each candidate. Once validated, the scores are calculated according the manual method of content analysis.

The software system generates four distinct classes of output: (1) an interlinear listing of each grammatical clause and the scores assigned to it; (2) a scoring summary for each content analysis scale including a comparison with established norms for each scale; (3) an analysis or interpretation of the scales score in textual form; and (4) possible neuropsychiatric diagnostic classifications take from the Diagnostic and Statistical Manual IV (DSM-IV) of the American Psychiatric Association that a clinician might consider in evaluating the patient.

The only information the computer program has regarding the patient is age, sex, ethnicity, educational level, and the verbal sample. Under ordinary circumstances, the user is expected to amplify the computer's assessment with any other pertinent data available.

METHODS AND PROCEDURES

The senior author of this study sees and treats a large group of outpatients with multiple sclerosis. Our goals in this research was to develop and test an alternative method of obtaining samples of a patient's speech during the neurologist's typical diagnostic and verbal behavior that has been generally used by some of us. These other therapeutic sessions, instead of employing other methods of eliciting methods include: (1) Having patients talk for five minutes on purposely ambiguous instructions to talk about any interesting or dramatic life experiences[2-4,11,12]; (2) Having subjects write verbal samples in response to ambiguous instructions[13] or other instructions, for example, in a study involving adolescents with an eating disorder in a residential treatment center were asked to write within one week of admission an answer to the question "How does your eating disorder affect you and what do you feel are the causes?" and "Have you improved over the past two weeks since you last wrote and why?"[14]; (3) Having subjects carry out conversations, for example, between physicians, nurses, and family members of a seriously ill patient[15]; (4) Scoring letters written by famous people, such as, Napoleon Bonaparte[16] or Mahatma Gandhi[17]; or written notes of a subject [Ted Kacynski, the Unabomber][18]; (5) scoring what a patient or subject was understood to say using only voice-recognition software[19,20].

In the present study, Dr. Stanley van den Noort carried out his usual method of clinically relating to his patient with multiple sclerosis, not infrequently with a family member present, and both his queries and comments were recorded as well as the patient's verbal responses. Dr. van den Noort's verbal comments were deleted from the transcriptions and only the patient's verbal responses were preserved, whether or not these verbalizations were fragmentary or incomplete since they were always in response to questions or comments from Dr. van den Noort. Identifying data related to the patient were eliminated, except for confidentially coded numbers, which were preserved for identification purposes.

The verbal responses of each patient were typed onto a computer diskette in Microsoft Word, and the typescript was converted to ASCII, which the computer software reads. Then each diskette was run on PCAD 2000[10] all the computerized scales. The software notes whether the score obtained on each scale is zero, one, two or three standard deviations different from the normative score for each scale. This information is made available to the user, either at the end of the summary of scores for each scale or on a spreadsheet showing summaries of the content analysis scores on all the scales scored.

RESULTS

Subjects

At this point, sixteen adult outpatients with multiple sclerosis have participated in this study. All of them have been receiving an auto-immune inhibiting drug. Table 1 provides two illustrations of the kind of verbal responses these patients give, and verbalizations which the artificial intelligence computer program analyzes.

Noteworthy from the Table 1A and 1B is that though the diagnostic and clinical assessment verbal contributions of the interviewer (Dr. Van den Noort) are omitted and only the verbal responses of the patients with multiple sclerosis are examined and scored by the computer program, these verbal activities in themselves, though sometimes fragmentary, convey meanings and cognitive and emotional empirical observations.

Table 1A. Examples of Verbal Responses

Name: 7
Race: White
Sex: Female
Age: 59
Education: 5 {one year of college}
Diagnosis: Multiple Sclerosis
There is probably more. Up to 250 of Baclofen. Still 59. Surgery. Mostly infertility. Not bad, not up until I had pre-eclampsia, then I always had high blood pressure. I was 36. Yes, first and only son. Never got off the medications. We had Kaiser insurance and I do not know why but it started to peak and go high and higher. Yes, 200/100. Another doctor found a combination to bring it down and now with all of the medications I am taking I do not know what it is now but basically that is the only thing. Approximately for 11 years, little startles in my leg, doctor gave me medicine and that went on for years like that and then it started during the day while driving. If I could keep my mind off from it, it did not last long and they would go away. One year ago this July, 2002, for spasms that I could not handle any more. I was on medicine for that. She gave me Flexaril and Clonapine and said if this works, then I will give you Cinamet thinking I had restless leg syndrome. Cinamet worked and I took it every 6 hours but then I just worked it down. Then she sent me to a neurologist, and they immediately started me on Baclofen. That was his associate, Dr. S. He said I need B12, that didn't work and he said I had strokes for 10 years and that was what causing the spasms. Then I went back to Dr. J. and he said I had MS. I was signed up for a Baclofen trial, no not a trial, a pump. Every 6 hours and initially that worked. They never told me to stop or to decrease the Baclofen. Then I talked to Joyce and she told me they generally do not use that much and so I quit. I do not remember a lot of what happened. I saw Dr. O. and he said I did not have MS. I found it to be very hard. Oh and I also have numbness in my toes and the balls of my feet. I am taking Neurontin for that. 300 mgs 3 X's a day. Thank goodness for the Cinamet. I am on that every 2 hours now and it is not working real well. No...I would say 1 a week. I am a bad girl. Clonapen and then Dr. O. said I was supposed to play with that. I take it but there is another mind altering thing and I take it at night to help me sleep. No. Shake. My father and my mother did shake. My mother had Parkinson's Disease and she was on L-Dopa. Oh fine, well I have only been taking it for one year so that is fine. Superintendent in insurance company. He is 23 years old.

Table 1B. Examples of Verbal Responses

Name: 6
Race: White
Sex: Female
Age: 40
Education: 6 {Registered Nurse}
Diagnosis: Multiple Sclerosis
Forty. I am an RN, BS. I did med-surg. At Hoag Hospital. My left leg started to get numb. And I had episodes of numbness before but usually they away and this just stayed. Maybe one year, on and off. Back in '95 when it came and stayed. And it just remained numb and I had a hard time walking on it and I went to see an orthopedic surgeon and he said I had like a disc thing so I went to physical therapy for a long time. Then my hands started getting numb. I said, wait now, something is wrong here. So I said I need to see a neurologist. So that is when I saw Dr. C. and she diagnosed me. That was in '95. Pretty much. I said when I went in there I have MS but Dr. C. said she did not like to make that diagnosis until I have some backing. Yes, I started Betaseron. I stayed on it for 2 years but then I started to get headaches and then I went on to Avonex. I guess that just works better for me. I had a baby in-between so I stopped taking it for awhile. No, I got pregnant on Avonex, I'm done with babies. Oh, how funny. I see Dr. F. H. She is in Huntington Beach. Very well. Just numbness in my left leg and I kinda have trouble walking. Occasionally. A year or so. SSI. Medicare. No medical history of anything. Not that I am aware of. Pasadena area. No medical history except MS. I had meningitis. They had an epidemic of meningitis at Hoag. I had a headache, I wanted to get off the floor, oh you need to go to the ER and get an LP. So I said all right, I went down there. They did a lumbar puncture and they got me up right after but I didn't care, I just wanted to go home. I got a spinal headache that was so bad, I thought I was going to die. Ever since then I have not felt normal or something. And I think some bacteria got into my back. I had to stay down, I could not get up. Oh, I thought it was a bad job. No problems with the bladder. Sometimes. Then it goes away. Left hand, is clumsy too. Once a week. Every couple of days or so. Black spot in my eye, a long time ago, '92. When I looked straight ahead, it was a large black spot, they diagnosed it as...I don't know. I have forgotten. About one week. I went to an ophthalmologist, and she said I was going blind. It just wore off. It wasn't a floater. There was an incident when I took the boards, I got so upset about it, I could not walk at all. That lasted for about a week or so. Never have seen a psychiatrist.

Table 2 shows the spreadsheet summarizing the number of standard deviations each patient deviated from the norm on each content analysis scale.

Table 2 provides a summary of the standard deviations from norms of the validated content analysis scales and their subscales derived from the computerized content analysis of the verbalizations of each of the multiple sclerotic patients. In spite of the fragmented and incomplete characteristics of these patient verbalizations, highly relevant objective perspectives and dimensions are recorded. Preoccupations with Sickness (elevated in 15 out of 16 patients) are notable. And among these elevated Sickness scores, Somatic Concerns (14 out of 16) are elevated. Various subtypes of elevated anxiety (Mutilation, Separation, and Guilt anxiety) are recognized among some patients. On the other hand, elevated Hostility Outward and Ambivalent Hostility (hostility direct to the speaker by others) does not occur; whereas, Hostility Inward (hostility directed to the self) occurs relatively frequently (6 out of 16 patients). And with respect to the dimensions of Human Relations, 11 out of 16 reveal significantly diminished scores. Likewise, with the dimension of Achievement Strivings, 6 out of 16 reveal significantly reduced scores. And not surprisingly 7 of the 16 reveal significantly decreased scores in the Quality of Life dimension.

Table 2. Deviations from norms on each scale for each subject

Subject	1	2	3	4	5	6	7	8	9	10	11	12	13	14	15	16
Death Anxiety	0	0	0	0	1	2	0	0	0	1	0	2	0	1	0	0
Mutilation Anxiety	1	0	1	0	0	1	0	1	1	1	1	0	1	1	0	0
Separation Anxiety	0	1	0	0	0	0	0	0	0	0	0	1	1	0	0	0
Guilt Anxiety	0	0	0	0	0	1	0	0	0	0	0	1	0	0	1	0
Shame Anxiety	0	0	0	0	0	0	0	0	0	0	0	0	0	0	0	0
Diffuse Anxiety	0	1	0	0	0	0	0	0	0	0	0	0	0	1	1	0
Total Anxiety	0	0	0	0	0	1	0	0	0	0	0	1	1	1	0	0
Hostility Out – Overt	0	0	0	0	0	0	0	0	0	0	0	0	0	0	0	0
Hostility Out – Covert	0	0	0	0	0	0	0	0	0	0	0	0	0	0	0	0
Total Hostility Out	0	0	0	0	0	0	0	0	0	0	0	0	0	0	0	0
Hostility Inward	1	0	0	0	0	1	1	0	0	0	0	1	1	2	0	0
Ambivalent Hostility	0	0	0	0	0	0	0	0	0	0	0	0	0	0	0	0
Schizophrenic	0	0	0	1	0	0	0	0	0	0	0	0	0	0	0	0
Cognitive Impairment	0	1	0	0	0	0	0	0	0	0	3	0	0	0	0	0
Hope	0	0	0	0	0	-1	0	0	0	0	0	0	0	0	0	0
Hopelessness	0	0	0	0	0	0	0	0	0	0	0	0	0	0	0	0
Self-Accusation	0	0	0	0	0	0	0	0	0	0	0	0	0	0	0	0
Psychomotor Retardation	0	0	0	0	0	0	0	0	0	0	0	0	0	0	0	0
Somatic Concerns	2	3	2	3	1	3	1	2	1	0	0	3	3	1	1	3
Death and Mutilation Depression	1	0	1	0	1	1	0	1	1	1	1	1	0	1	0	0
Separation Depression	0	0	0	0	0	0	0	0	0	0	0	0	0	0	0	0
Hostility Directed Outward	0	0	0	0	0	0	0	0	0	0	0	0	0	0	0	0
Total Depression	1	0	0	0	0	1	0	0	0	0	0	1	0	1	0	0
Health	0	0	0	1	0	0	0	0	0	0	0	0	3	1	0	0
Sickness	3	3	3	3	3	3	2	3	3	2	2	3	3	3	3	3
Health/Sickness	2	3	1	3	1	2	0	1	1	1	1	2	3	3	1	3
Human Relations	-1	-1	0	-1	-1	-1	-1	-1	-1	0	0	0	-1	-2	0	-1
Support	0	0	0	0	0	0	0	0	0	0	0	0	0	0	0	0
Deterrents	1	2	2	0	1	3	0	0	0	0	0	2	0	1	0	1
Achievement Strivings	-1	-1	0	-1	0	-2	0	0	0	0	0	-1	0	0	0	-2
Dependency Strivings	0	0	0	0	0	0	0	0	0	0	0	0	0	0	0	0
Frustrated Dependency	0	0	0	0	0	0	0	0	0	0	0	0	0	0	0	0
Quality of Life	-1	0	0	-1	-1	-1	0	0	0	-1	0	-1	0	-2	0	0

Multiple sclerosis in early stages of the disease may have notable cognitive function, and only two of these 16 patients have significantly elevated scores in cognitive impairment.

Most of the group of patients were being administered a psychoactive drug, such as a tranquilizer, antidepressant, and/or anti-anxiety agent and such medicaments do, indeed, suppress and inhibit the usually depressing and anxiety producing effects of multiple sclerosis and it disabling consequences and course. So our findings with regards to the magnitude of these mentally disabling concomitants of the disorder are probably minimized to some extent by the neuropsychopharmacological agents[7].

DISCUSSION

The technological advances occurring in our society will, hopefully, have increasing beneficial effects of the diagnosis, course, and treatment of serious, crippling, and fatal diseases. Multiple sclerosis and other auto-immune disorders, various kinds of cancer, diabetes mellitus, Parkinson's disease, Alzheimer's disease and other dimentias, cardiovascular disorders, aging itself, provide continuing challenges to medical sciences.

Objectively, recording the courses of these disorders is another challenge and stimulus for application of our developing informatics and computer sciences. This report constitutes another step in the direction of such technological applications. In this report we have demonstrated that the computerized content analysis of a recorded transcript of a clinical interview by an expert neurologist of a group of 16 patients suffering from various stages of the auto-immune disease of multiple sclerosis can provide an objective measurement and perspective of the current mental and physical status of each patient.

Many previous publications involving the use of this computerized content analysis methodology have demonstrated that under a variety of circumstances such useful measurements can be made. The circumstances and situations originated with the use of five-minute speech samples elicited by purposely ambiguous standard instructions to talk about any interesting or dramatic life experiences. Subsequently, the measurement of similar neuropsychobiological dimensions from conversations and verbal text has been demonstrated to be possible, valid, and fruitful.

REFERENCES

[1] American Psychiatric Association, Diagnostic and Statistical Manual of Mental Disorders (DSM IV). (1994). 4th Edition. Washington, DC, USA.

[2] Gottschalk, L.A., and Gleser, G.C. (1969). The Measurement of Psychological States from the Content Analysis of Verbal Behavior. Los Angeles, Berkeley, USA: University of California Press.

[3] Gottschalk, L.A., Winget, C.N., Gleser, G.C. (1969). *Manual of Instructions for Using the Gottschalk-Gleser Content Analysis Scales: Anxiety, Hostility, and Social Alienation-Personal Disorganization.* Los Angeles, Berkeley: University of California Press.

[4] Gottschalk, L.A. (Ed.) *The Content Analysis of Verbal Behavior*. Further Studies. New York, USA: Spectrum Publications, 1979.

[5] Bechtel, R.J. (1997). *Developments in computer science with applications to text analysis.* In: Roberts CW (Ed.) Text Analysis for the Social Sciences. Mahway, New Jersey, USA: Erlbaum, pp. 239-250.

[6] Gottschalk, L.A. (1995). *Content Analysis of Verbal Behavior*. New Findings and

Clinical Applications. Hillsdale, New Jersey, USA: Lawrence Erlbaum Publishers.

[7] Gottschalk, L.A. (1999). The application of a computerized measurement of the content analysis of natural language to the assessment of psychoactive drugs. *Methods and Findings in Experimental and Clinical Pharmacology*, 21, 133-135.

[8] Gottschalk, L.A., Bechtel, R.J. (1982). The measurement of anxiety through the content analysis of verbal samples. *Comprehensive Psychiatry*, 23, 364-369.

[9] Gottschalk, L.A., Bechtel, R.J. (1995). Computerized measurement of the content analysis of natural language. *Computer Methods and Programs in Biomedicine*, 47, 123-130.

[10] Gottschalk, L.A., Bechtel, R.J. (1998-2002). PCAD 2000: Psychiatric Content Analysis and Diagnosis. Corona del Mar, CA, USA: GB Software.

[11] Lebovitz, A.H., and Holland, J.C. (1983). Use of the Gottschalk-Gleser verbal content analysis scales with medically ill patients. *Psychosomatic Medicine*, 45, 305-320.

[12] Koch, U., Schofer, G. (Eds.) (1986). Sprachinhalstanalyse in der psychosomatischen und psychiatrischen forschung. Grundlagen und Anwenduggssstudien mit den Affekstkalen von Gottschalk und Gleser. Weinheim, Germany: Psychologie Verlag Union.

[13] Lavid, N.R., Grayden, T.J., Gottschalk, L.A., Bechtel, R.J. (2002). Computerized assessment of the enforced hospitalization and medication from the notes of hospitalized psychiatric patients. *American Journal of Forensic Psychiatry*, 23, 55-69.

[14] Reynolds, W.M., Gottschalk, L.A., Bechtel, R.J. (2000). *Psychiatric Content Analysis and Diagnosis*. In: Plake, B.S., Impara, J.C., Murphy, L.L. (Eds.) The Fourteenth Mental Measurements Yearbook. Lincoln, NE, USA: University of Nebraska Press, pp. 966-968.

[15] Gottschalk, L.A., Bechtel, R.J., Buchman, T.G., Ray, S.E. (2003). A computerized measure of quality of life derived from the content analysis of natural language. *Research Communications in Biological Psychology and Psychiatry*, 27, 3-14.

[16] Gottschalk, L.A., DeFrancisco, D., Bechtel, R.J. (2002). Computerized content analysis of some adolescent letters of Napoleon Bonaparte: a test of the validity of the method. *Journal of Nervous and Mental Disease*, 199, 542-548.

[17] Gottschalk, L.A., Bechtel, R.J. (2005). Computerized content analysis of the writings of Mahatma Gandhi. (In press) *Journal of Nervous and Mental Disease*.

[18] Gottschalk, L.A., Gottschalk, L.H. (1999). Computerized content analysis of the Unabomber's writings. *American Journal of Forensic Psychiatry*, 20, 5-31.

[19] Lavid, N.E., Gottschalk, L.A., Bechtel, R.J., Gormanm, J., Brown, A., LeDay, R. (2005). Computerized measurement of the neuropsychiatric traits in adolescents with eating disorder. (In press) In: Eating Disorders. Nova Science Publishers.

[20] Gottschalk, L.A. (1999). The application of a computerized measurement of the content analysis of natural language to the assessment of the effects of psychoactive drugs. *Methods and Findings in Experimental and Clinical Pharmacology*, 21, 133-135.

[21] Gottschalk, L.A., Hoigaard-Martin, J. (1986). A depression scale applicable to verbal samples. *Psychiatry Research*, 17, 213-2276.

[22] Gottschalk, L.A., Bechtel, R.J. (2004). Computerized psychodynamic diagnosis and psychotherapy. Presented at the Annual Meeting of the American Association for Artificial Intelligence. Washington, DC, USA.

In: Multiple Sclerosis Research Progress
Editors: H. Schwarz, L. Walter ISBN: 978-1-60456-570-6
© 2008 Nova Science Publishers, Inc.

Chapter 6

CD30 MOLECULE, THE IMMUNE SYSTEM AND MULTIPLE SCLEROSIS

Anna Maria Berghella[1], Patrizia Pellegrini, Ida Contasta, Antonio Carolei* and Domenico Adorno
Istituto CNR per i Trapianti d'Organo e l'Immunocitologia (ITOI) L'Aquila, Italia
*Dipartimento di Neurologia dell'Università dell'Aquila, Italia

ABSTRACT

Objectives

On the basis of our own and other research on the CD30 molecule, we hypothesized that CD30 may be the unknown molecule involved in the cell contact-dependent suppression of T regulatory cells (Trs) by regulatory dendritic cells (rDCs). Trs are responsible for maintaining the physiological balance between TH1/TH2/TH3 immune responses and central and peripheral tolerance. Thus DC CD30-mediated signals are of key importance both in the initial phase of immune response as well as in maintaining the physiological balance between TH1/TH2/TH3 immune responses. We believe that abnormal CD30 signalling can lead to the generation of autoimmune diseases such as multiple sclerosis (MS) and hence, in addition to substantiating the hypothesis above, our objective was also to clarify the immunopathological mechanisms involved in MS and the causes of immunosuppressive drug failure.

Methods

We determined network interactions between sCD30, sBcl2 and TH1/TH2/TH3 cytokines (IL12p70, IL12p40, IL10 and TGFβ) in immature (I) DC and DC culture

[1] Corresponding author: Berghella Anna Maria, Tel: +39.0862.27129 Fax: +39.0862.410758. E-mail address: a.berghella@itoi.cnr.it

supernatants in IFNβ–1a treated and untreated relapsing-remitting MS (RRMS) patients. TH1/TH2/TH3 cytokine networks in whole blood culture supernatants in PHA activation conditions were also studied.

Results

Our overall results, in support of our hypothesis, indicate that CD30 is involved in the cell contact-dependent suppression of TH cells by regulatory IDCs (rIDCs), and rDCs and that this contact-dependent suppression is indispensable for the generation of TGFβ producing Tr (TH3) subsets. Alterations at this level were found in untreated patients, while IFNβ–1a treatment was found to restore the physiological mechanisms by increasing suppressive (sp-) IDC and sp-DC activity (IL10) resulting in a lowering of sCD30 levels, re-establishment of CD30-mediated signals and equilibrium between type1- and type2-like immune response (rICD1/rIDC2 and rDC1/rDC2). Consequently, CD30 being responsible for the balance between Tr1/Tr2, re-establishes equilibrium between immune responses and central and peripheral tolerance. However, it also appears that IFNβ–1a treatment is responsible for the *in vivo* suppression of patient TH1-DC functions which involve the induction of Tr1s for the deletion of self aggressive cells in the immune response in activation conditions, and this may explain the cause of immunosuppressive drug failure.

Conclusion

CD30 mediates signals for a key mechanism involving dendritic and T regulatory cells responsible for maintaining the physiological balance between immune responses and central and peripheral tolerance. Multiple sclerosis is the result of alterations at this level; however, IFNβ-1a treatment is partially successful in restoring the physiological mechanisms affected. Further study can lead to new ways of identifying methods for more effective prevention and treatment of immunopathological conditions such as autoimmune diseases, transplant rejection, allergy and tumor.

Key Words: CD30 molecule, Dendritic and T regulatory cells, peripheral and central immune tolerance, multiple sclerosis, IFNβ-1a treatment, immunotherapy

INTRODUCTION

The CD30 antigen, a member of the TNF receptor superfamily [1-3], was originally identified as a cell surface antigen on primary and cultured Hodgkin's and Reed-Sternberg cells [4,5]. CD30 is also expressed in several virally transformed T and B cell lines [5,6]. Normal PBMCs do not express CD30 but a subset of CD45RO+ T lymphocytes, the memory cells, express CD30 after mitogenic stimulation [7,8]. This is an important finding in autoimmunity research because CD30 can hence be used as a marker for self-reactive cells [9].

The function of CD30 in mature peripheral T lymphocytes is unclear, but there is evidence that CD30 can act as a signal transduction molecule [10-16]. Furthermore, CD30 and its physiological ligand (CD30L) are expressed on activated T cells, neutrophils, eosinophils and resting B cells [17, 18]. Ligation of CD30 by an anti-CD30mAb (CD30L) leads to the rapid activation of NF-KB (linked to cell survival) in T cells [14] mediated through a TNFR-associated factor (TRAF) 2 and TRAF5 [15, 16], whereas cross-linking of CD30 with an antagonistic mAb (anti-CD30L) increases the levels of Ca++ [19] in T cells.

Signalling through CD30 was found to promote the development of TH2 cells [20] and CD30 is generally used as a marker for TH2 cell populations [21-23]. However, the results of previous studies [24-26] lead us to believe that CD30 is a marker for an important subpopulation of immunoregulatory cells responsible for the balance between TH1/TH2 type responses.

Classically immune responses have been classified into type1, which provides cell-mediated immune response, and type2, which supports B helper function and the humoral immune response. [27]. These responses are regulated by the TH1 and TH2 subsets of CD4+ T helper cells respectively. Although both subsets produce IL-3, GMCSF and TNF-α, only TH1 cells produce IL-2, IFN-γ [28], whilst TH2 cells produce other cytokines, such as IL-4, IL-5, IL-6, and IL-10 [29].

The polarization of the immune response into TH1 or TH2 cellular types is not absolute and the ratio of these cells varies according to physiological demand and clinical conditions [30]. *In vivo* and *in vitro* studies in mice have demonstrated that cytokines play a crucial role in maintaining balance in the development of T cells into TH1 or TH2 types [31], and pathological conditions were found to arise from abnormalities in the balance between the production of TH1 and TH2 cytokines [32]. It seems that the relative proportion of each cell type depends on the environmental cytokines present during activation [33].

IFNγ induces the proliferation of TH1 cells [34] whilst IL-4 was shown to be essential for the development of TH2 cells [35] and to inhibit the differentiation of precursors into TH1 cells [36]. IL-10 is an important physiological regulator of inflammatory and immune responses [37], and its *in vivo* production is associated with TH2-like responses; it is a more powerful inhibitor of IFNγ, macrophages and TH1 functions than IL-4 [34,38] and so is produced when its inhibiting activities favour homeostasis. Alterations in IL10 levels cause an imbalance in the network which can have profound pathological consequences [39-41]. IL12p40, a homodimer, also promotes TH2 immunity by acting as an IL12 antagonist [42,43] whilst IL12p70, a heterodimer, is a major TH1/driving cytokine promoting cell-mediated immunity.

More recently, an additional regulatory CD4+ T-cell subset was identified, designated TH3, and is characterized by the production of TGFβ [44]. These cells are involved in the regulation of TH1 and TH2 functions and there is now increased effort being made to understand the mechanisms of TGFβ-mediated immunological suppression and/or stimulation [44]. TGFβ is thought to function as a differentiation switch, counteracting existing differentiation programs of cells as they pass from one stage of differentiation to the next.

Consequently, network interactions between TH1/TH2/TH3 cytokines, which together are believed to control the polarization of TH cells into TH1 or TH2 or TH3 types (and so the type of physiological immune response), need to be studied carefully as disturbances in this network can result in disease [45]. Network interactions between TH1/TH2/TH3 cytokines in serum are studied to evaluate the influence of cell environment on TH polarization, whilst network interactions between TH1/TH2/TH3 cytokines produced by immunological cells are studied to establish functional type (TH1 or TH2 or TH3). Experiments under physiological conditions allow us to study the resting conditions of the immune response; while those with activation stimuli (specific to the immunological situations in study), show us the activation characteristics of the immune responses.

To confirm our hypothesis that CD30 is a marker for an important subpopulation of immunoregulatory cells responsible for the balance between TH1/TH2 type responses, we looked at network interactions between soluble CD30 (sCD30, a marker of CD30 expression), sBcl2 (a marker of cell survival), and TH1/TH2 cytokines in peripheral whole blood cultures of healthy subjects [46]. Our line of thinking was confirmed when we found that CD30 signals trigger functional mechanisms responsible for changes in the levels of production of several important TH1 and TH2 cytokines involved in the regulation of the physiological balance between TH1/TH2 functions [46]. Our results also showed a lack of normal CD30 immunoregulatory activity when the interaction between CD30 molecule and its ligand (CD30/CD30L) had been blocked or when IL4 or IFNγ activity had been blocked by monoclonal antibodies.

The expression and function of CD30 molecule on DCs, on the other hand, was still unclear [47,48]. On the basis of our previous CD30 research we hypothesized that CD30-mediated signals on DCs may also have an important role in the regulation of the physiological balance between TH1/TH2 immune responses.

We studied this situation in RRMS patients since it was found that DC phenotype and function are altered in MS patients, implying TH1-biased responses [49-52]. Consequently, by comparing IFNβ–1a treated and untreated patients, we were able to clarify the physiological mechanisms involved in DC CD30-mediated signals and MS.

RRMS patients suffer acute attacks followed by a variable recovery period. During the attack, inflammation results in injury to the myelin sheaths, the oligodendrocytes and, to a lesser extent, the axons and nerve cells themselves [53-56]. However, the efficacy of IFNβ in the treatment of RRMS is well established [57]; it reduces the frequency and severity of relapses and delays progression of neurological disability [58-62]. IFNβ is available in two forms for MS therapy: IFNβ–1a, which is structurally identical to native human IFNβ and IFNβ–1b which differs from the native protein both in its sequence and lack of glycosilation. Glycosilation is important as it provides greater stability and may be important in receptor recognition and binding [57]. We chose IFNβ–1a treated patients because the structure of IFNβ–1a results in a 10-15 fold higher specific activity compared with IFNβ–1b [63].This study [64] confirmed the role of DC CD30 in the regulation of the physiological balance between TH1/TH2 immune responses: abnormal increases in sCD30 levels produced a disruption of the DC CD30-mediated signals. Additionally, IFNβ–1a treatment was found to modify patient immune response by inducing mechanisms determining a fall in sCD30 levels and leading to a partial re-establishment of IDC and DC regulation of TH1/TH2 immune response balance.

Hence we concluded that an abnormal increase in the levels of sCD30 can also produce an imbalance between TH1/TH2 functions. In support of these findings are the results of other researchers showing that sCD30 binds to CD30 on the cell membrane with high affinity blocking transmembrane signalling by CD30 molecule [65]; sCD30 levels have also found to be a prediction factor for immunological risks [66,67].

Overall our previous CD30 study indicates that a disregulation in TH1 and/or TH2 cytokines, or an inhibition of CD30/CD30L interaction or an abnormal increase in sCD30 levels is responsible for a lack of normal CD30 immunoregulation and the consequences of this could be immunopathological conditions, such as inappropriate TH cellular generation of TH1 cytotoxic lymphocytes and/or TH2 suppressive cells.

However a lack of Trs (TH3) could also be a consequence of the above, since it has recently become clear that DCs play an essential role in inducing and modulating Trs and there is increasing evidence that normal Trs also exert regulatory function [68], thereby preventing or limiting autoimmune disease, by suppressing self-reactive T-cells. CD30 signalling was found, in fact, to protect against autoimmunity by limiting the proliferative potential of self-reactive cells, whilst a disruption of this regulation due to the absence of CD30 signalling results in the activation of self-reactive cells, rather than deletion [9,69,70]. Eradication of Trs was found to result in the development of various autoimmune diseases indicating that the main function of Trs is the suppression of pathological self-reactive T cell responses [71]. Furthermore, in MS it is widely accepted that self-reactive T-cells are key mediators of the auto-immune mechanisms and that these cells are T-antigen-primed cells, which cross the blood-brain barrier into the central nervous system and re-encounter T-antigens setting-up a pro-inflammatory loop which leads to injury of axons and glia [72].

MS is considered an autoimmune disease that is induced when T Helper 1 (TH1) cells recognize components of the myelin sheath. Activated, self-reactive T cells within lesions are believed to drive the chronic inflammatory process and activate local or hematogeneous macrophages that destroy myelin [73]. Within actively demyelinating lesions, TH1-related cytokines such as IFNγ, TNFα or IL2, are expressed by invading leukocytes and local glial cells [74]. The spectrum of chemokines and chemokine receptors observed, is also consistent with a TH1-driven inflammatory response [75].

Furthermore, the transfer of suppressive activity from rDCs to Trs would appear to be mediated through cell-cell contact, but the molecule involved in this cell contact-dependent suppression is still largely unknown.

It is well known that the immune system, a highly effective and dynamic cellular network, must be able to distinguish harmful from innocuous foreign antigens and self from non-self structures to prevent both unessential and self-reactive immune responses. However, there is an innate risk of the development of self-reactive T-cells, given the process of T cell receptor generation based on random rearrangements and promiscuity of the resulting receptors [76]. To maintain tolerance against self as well as protective immunity against pathogens, a sophisticated and highly balanced immune mechanism has evolved for generation of antigen-specific tolerance induction. The induction of this antigen-specific T cell tolerance and its maintenance in the periphery are critical for preventing self-reactive immune responses.

It is, furthermore, well known that tolerance induction based on clonal deletion of self-reactive T cells in the thymus, upon interaction with DC, is a mechanism to prevent self-reactive immune reactions in the periphery, and is defined as central tolerance [77]. However, clonal deletion of self-reactive T cells is incomplete because detectable number of self-reactive T cells escapes central deletion and reach the periphery. Therefore, additional systems for tolerance induction and maintenance must be present in the periphery [78]. These mechanisms of peripheral tolerance include DC induction of populations of Trs.

Several lines of evidence indicate that Trs cells arise in the thymus upon interaction with medullary DCs during a process of negative selections (this process can be regarded as the "third function" of the thymus) [78] and then emigrate from the thymus to populate the periphery [79]. There are two broad categories of Trs: one category consists of naturally occurring Trs that emigrate from the thymus, are present in the circulation of healthy individuals and require the expression of the cytotoxic T lymphocyte antigen 4 (CTLA-4) and or glucocorticoid-induced tumor necrosis factor receptor (GITR). These Trs act in a cytokine–independent, antigen-non specific, manner and appear to require cell-to-cell interaction with rDCs to receive suppressive activity, and with conventional TH cells to induce suppressive activity in new Trs. The second category includes Trs, TH3 cells and sp-Trs, that inhibit normal CD4+ TH reactivity via the production and release of the immunomodulatory cytokines TGFβ and IL10 respectively [80, 81]. The main mechanism of suppression seems to be the inhibition of IL2 transcription in the responder T cell population [82].

In *in vitro* studies on cell membrane molecule expression, Trs have been identified as CD4+ CD25+ T cells in rats and humans [83-86] and in both species have a memory phenotype (CD45RO+ in humans) indicating that these cells have previously encountered antigens *in vivo*. Human and mouse Trs cells have increased expression of the putative regulatory marker CTLA-4 [81,83,84,87-90] and GITR [91].

However, despite the extensive phenotypic analysis, none of the markers described above are exclusively expressed by rDCs or Trs. Furthermore, the transfer of suppressive activity from rDCs to Trs is mediated through cell-cell contact, but the molecules involved in this cell contact-dependent suppression are still largely unknown [92].

On the basis of the above considerations, the aim of this work was to substantiate our hypothesis that CD30 costimulator molecule is in fact the unknown molecule involved in the cell contact-dependent suppression of Trs by rDCs. We believe that abnormal CD30 signalling can lead to the generation of autoimmune diseases such as MS and hence, in substantiating our hypothesis above, our objective was also to clarify the immunopathological mechanisms involved in MS and the causes of immunosuppressive drug failure.

Hence we studied the functional-dynamic cellular networks (F-dynamic networks) of IDC/rIDCs/Trs, and DC/rDCs/Trs by determining: network interactions between sCD30, sBcl2 and TH1/TH2/TH3 cytokines (IL12p70, IL12p40, IL10 and TGFβ) in IDC, DC and whole blood culture supernatants in IFNβ–1a treated and untreated RRMS patients. IL10 and TGFβ are well-known rDCs and Trs immunomodulatory factors [93,94]. IL12p70, a heterodimer, is a major TH1/driving cytokine promoting cell-mediated immunity. In contrast, IL12p40, a homodimer, does not mediate IL12 activity but acts as an IL12 antagonist [42,43] and so has an anti-TH1 function, promoting TH2 immunity

Patients and Methods

Patients

The study was approved by the local Ethics Committee and all persons gave their informed consent prior to their inclusion in the study.

We investigated 34 patients with clinically defined RRMS admitted to the MS Center of the Department of Neurology of the University of L'Aquila. None of the patients had suffered an exacerbation in the 3 months before entry into the study, received corticosteroids in the month prior to entry, or immunosuppressants in the previous 6 months. The Expanded Disability Status Scale (EDSS) was used as a clinical parameter. We considered the absence of clinical relapses for at least 3 months as a marker of disease inactivity.

The treated group consisted of 3 men and 13 women, with a mean age ±SE of 32.3 ± 1.9 years and a mean EDSS score±SE of 2 ± 0.3. They had been receiving IFNβ–1a treatment [22μg (4 patients) or 44μg (12 patients)] subcutaneously trice-weekly for a mean period±SE of 27.5 ± 1.4 months (range: 2 to 60 months). The untreated group of patients, matched for sex age and EDSS score consisted of 7 men and 11 women with a mean age±SE of 34.7± 2.6 and a mean EDSS score±SE of 2 ± 0.2.

We also considered: time since last treatment (TLT), treatment duration (TD) and patient age. TLT was 1 day in 4 patients and 2 days in 12. TD was 2 to 7 months in 4 patients, 8 to 36 months in 7 patients, and 37 to 60 months in 5 patients.

Patient groups for TLT, TD and different dose were matched for sex, age and EDSS score.

This is a paired samples study since sCD30, sBcl2 and TH1/TH2/TH3 cytokine levels were determined in IDC and DC culture supernatants (with and without stimuli) for each patient sample; TH1/TH2/TH3 cytokine levels in whole blood culture supernatants with PHA stimulus (T cells) were also evaluated.

PBMC Separation and Generation of Dendritic Cells (DCs) from Monocytes

A sample of heparinized blood (20 IU/ml blood - Liquemin-Roche) was taken from each subject and diluted 1:4 with medium at room temperature. PBMCs were separated by centrifugation (160 g for 20 minutes at 20°C) over a Lymphoprep gradient (Nycomed Norvay). PBMCs were recovered from plasma/Lymphoprep interface, washed three times with medium (200 g for 10 minutes at 20°C).

Monocytes from PBMC samples were obtained by removing T cells, B cells, NK cells and granulocytes (if present): antibody mix was added to the PBMC sample and then depletion Dynabeads were added to capture the antibody bound cells. Dynabeads are uniform, supermagnetic, polystyrene beads coated with a Fc specific human IgG4 antibody against mouse IgG. The antibody mix contained a mixture of mouse monoclonal antibody for CD2, CD7, CD16 (specific for CD16a and CD16b), CD19 and CD56. The blocking reagent was gamma globulin to block FcR on monocytes. These coated cells were then separated with a magnet (Dynal MPC) and discarded. PBMCs were then transferred into a 15 ml tube, washed three times with PBS by centrifugation (at 225 g for 8 minutes at 2-8°C) and then re-suspended at $1x10^7$ per 100-200 μl PBS. 22 μl of blocking reagent and 20 μl of antibody mix for each $1x10^7$ MNC cells were added and incubated for 10 minutes at 2-8°C. The cells were washed (by adding 1 ml of PBS per $1x10^7$ MNC and centrifugation for 8 minutes at 500 g) and re-suspended in 0.9 ml of PBS per $1x10^7$ MNC. 100 μl of Depletion Dynabeads per $1x10^7$ MNC was added and incubated for 15 minutes at 2-8°C with gentle tilting and rotation. The total volume for cell and bead incubation should be 1 ml per $1x10^7$ MNC. The rosettes were re-suspended by careful pipetting 5-6 times before increasing the volume by adding 1-2 ml of PBS and placed in the Dynal Magnetic particle concentrator for 2 minutes. Isolated monocytes recovered were >98% viable and free of surface bound antibody or Dynabeads. Monocytes were re-suspended in RPMI 1640 (Sigma, endotoxin tested) complete medium containing 10% of AB male human serum (heat-inactivated for 30 minutes at 56°C), penicillin (50 UI/ml), streptomycin (50 μg/ml) and L-glutamine (0.2 mM).

The cells were incubated in 24-well plates at a concentration of 200.000 cells per ml at 37 °C in a humidified atmosphere of 5% CO_2 for 8 days and stimulated with 30 ng/ml of recombinant IL4 (Preprotech-England, specific activity of $>5x10^6$ U/mg), 30 ng/ml of recombinant GM-CSF (Preprotech-England, specific activity of $>1x10^7$ U/mg). On day 3, IL4 and GM-CSF were added again and on day 6, immature DCs were obtained. Immature DCs were stimulated with 100 μg/ml of LPS (Sigma), 0.1 ng/ml of recombinant human IFNβ (Preprotech-England, specific activity of $>2x10^7$ U/mg), 1000U/ml of recombinant human IFNγ (Collaborative Research incorporated, biomedical products, Bedford, Mass, specific activity 500.000 Units/100 μl) and DCs without stimuli were also prepared. After 2 days of culture the supernatant was removed from each well, centrifuged at 250 g and stored frozen in aliquots at –80°C until used.

Whole Blood Cell Cultures

The whole blood culture method [95-97] was used for the network study as it reflects, *in vivo* physiological conditions more accurately.

A 15 ml sample of heparinized blood (20 IU heparin/ml blood - Liquemin-Roche) was taken from each patient, and the samples, kept at room temperature, were used immediately. Venous blood was diluted 1:10 with RPMI-1640 medium (Sigma, endotoxin tested), which was supplemented with 0.2 mM of L-glutamine, 50 IU/ml of penicillin, 50 μg/ml streptomycin (Sigma) and 10% of human AB serum. Aliquots at $1x10^6$ cells were distributed in 12 mm polypropylene tubes. 10μg/ml of PHA (Sigma) was used for stimulation.

After 3 days of culture the supernatant was removed and cytokine levels determined.

The effect of adding heparin, which prevents clotting in whole blood cultures, was tested.

Cytokine Detection

Cytokine levels were determined using a solid phase sandwich Enzyme Linked-Immuno-Sorbent Assay (ELISA). ELISA assays are employed for the *in vitro* quantitative determination of cytokines and soluble molecules in cell culture medium [98]. Briefly, a monoclonal antibody specific for cytokine detection is coated into the wells of the microtiter strips. Samples (assayed in replicate), including standards of known and unknown cytokine concentrations, are pipetted into these wells. During the first incubation, the cytokine antigens are added to the wells. After washing, a biotinylated monoclonal antibody specific for the cytokine is incubated. Then the enzyme streptavidin-peroxidase is added. After incubation and washing to remove all unbound enzyme, a substrate solution, which acts on the bound enzyme, is added to induce a coloured reaction product. The intensity of this coloured product is directly proportional to the concentration of the cytokine present in the sample. A blood sample is taken from each subject and assayed for all cytokines. Thus all cytokines are determined in all patients. For intra-assay precision, samples of known cytokine concentration are assayed in replicates of 10 to determine precision within an assay, the coefficient of variation is <10%. For inter-assay precision, samples are assayed 30 times in multiple assays to determine precision between assays, the coefficient of variation is <10%.

The sensitivity of these ELISA assay was as follows: IL10 <1pg/ml, TGFβ1 <1.9pg/ml, IL2 <10pg/ml, IFNγ <5pg/ml, IL6 <2pg/ml, (Euroclone), IL12p40 <15pg/ml, IL12p70 <0.5 pg/ml, IL4<0.13 pg/ml (R&D System), sCD30<0.5 U/ml, sBcl2<1 U/ml (Bender Medsystem).

Data Analysis

Many recent advances in TH1/TH2/TH3 cytokine network research in MS have relied on the isolation of single cytokines using *in vitro* experiments with individual cell types and purified cytokines, or *in vivo* models using mice lacking the cytokine in question through the targeted destruction of the cytokine gene. These experimental approaches have been extremely successful in determining the influence of individual TH1 or TH2 or TH3 cytokines, but they do not allow a true assessment of the relative importance of each cytokine in the physiological network where all cytokines are functioning simultaneously. There is now an increasing need to understand how the immune system functions as a whole in order to understand more fully the development of pathological conditions such as autoimmunity, and in order to make immunological indices for more effective strategies to prevent and treat these pathologies. Currently the only way of studying the whole integrated system would appear to be through mathematical modelling and so, in addition to the study of statistical differences using the Wilcoxon rank test for paired samples, the Mann-Whitney U-test or Student's t-test as appropriate, multivariate statistical analyses -correlation, covariance and principal component analyses- were also carried out (using "Statgraphics software systems, full system 5.25 version 4.0" Graphics system by statistical graphics corporation ed. USA. 1989). Values of $p \leq 0.05$ were considered significant.

The procedure that analyses the correlation between parameters provides us with a matrix of coefficients of correlation (that vary from –1 to +1) and significance (p), and gives the degree of correlation between parameters within the network at any one moment in time. A positive correlation indicates that the parameters vary in the same direction, while negative correlation indicates that the parameters vary in the opposite direction. Statistically independent parameters have an expected correlation of zero.

The covariance analysis produce a matrix of covariance coefficients between parameters which can be positive or negative and which, in contrast to the correlation study, allows a dynamic analysis of how network components vary in respect to one another in any one moment of time. In fact, the covariance method measures the linear association between parameters and if parameters increase or decrease at the same time, the covariance is positive, whilst other changes are considered negative.

The principal component analysis plots the vectors of interaction between parameters within the network. The angle between vectors is inversely proportional to the correlation between them, the same vector direction indicates a positive correlation, the opposite vector direction indicates a negative correlation. This allows for a visualization of the situation under examination.

RESULTS

We report the levels of sCD30 and TH1/TH2/TH3 cytokines in IDC and DC culture supernatants and the levels of TH1/TH2/TH3 cytokines in whole blood culture supernatants as well as network interactions between IDC and DC sCD30, sBcl2 and TH1/TH2/TH3 cytokines, in relation to treatment.

Levels of sCD30 and TH1/TH2/TH3 Cytokines in IDC and DC Culture Supernatants and Levels of TH1/TH2/TH3 Cytokines in Whole Blood Culture Supernatants, in Treated and Untreated Groups

These results are detailed in Tables 1 and 2. Significantly higher (↑) values of IL10 (sp-DC) were found in the IDC-IFNβ supernatants of treated patients, while levels of IL12p70 were higher (TH1) in the IDC, IDC-IFNβ and IDC-IFNγ supernatants of untreated patients (Table 1). Levels of sCD30 in supernatants of IDC (resting immune response) and IDC-LPS (activated immune response) supernatants were also higher in untreated patients (MS disruption of CD30-mediated signals in resting and immune activated conditions).

Levels of IL12p70, IL12p40 and IL10 were significantly higher in IDC-LPS supernatants than in IDC supernatants (TH1/TH2 balance) in the treated group (Table 1). In the untreated group, levels of IL10 and IL12p40, but not IL12p70, were significantly higher in IDC-LPS supernatants than in IDC supernatants (TH1 disruption in activation conditions).

By comparing cytokine levels in whole blood supernatants we found higher levels of IFNγ in the PBMC-PHA supernatants of untreated patients whilst higher levels of IL4 were found in the PBMC supernatants of treated patients (Table 2). Furthermore, in treated patients PHA-IL10 levels were positively correlated to PHA-TGFβ, -IL4, -IL12p70, and -IFNγ ($r=0.5$ $p=0.045$, $r=0.5$ $p=0.042$, $r=0.5$ $p=0.05$ and $r=0.8$ $p<0.00001$ respectively), PHA-IFNγ levels were positively correlated to PHA-TGFβ, and -IL4 ($r=0.5$ $p=0.040$ and $r=0.6$ $p=0.01$ respectively) and PHA-IL4 levels were positively correlated to PHA-IL12p40 ($r=0.5$ $p=0.03$). In untreated patients, PHA-IL10 levels were positively correlated to PHA-IFNγ, -IL2, -IL4 and -IL12p40 ($r=0.7$ $p=0.0005$, $r=0.6$ $p=0.012$, $r=0.6$ $p=0.006$ and $r=0.5$ $p=0.034$ respectively), PHA-IFNγ levels were positively correlated to PHA-IL6, -IL2, -IL4 and -IL12p40 ($r=0.7$ $p=0.001$, $r=0.6$ $p=0.017$, $r=0.6$ $p=0.016$ and $r=0.8$ $p=0.002$ respectively) and PHA-IL4 and PHA-IL6 levels were positively correlated to PHA-IL12p40 levels ($r=0.6$ $p=0.011$, $r=0.6$ $p=0.028$ respectively).

In treated patients the EDDS parameter was correlated negatively to the levels of IDC TGFβ ($r= -0.7$ $p=0.02$), IDC-LPS TGFβ, IL12p70, IL12p40 ($r= -0.5$ $p=0.03$, $r= -0.6$ $p=0.006$ and $r= -0.5$ $p=0.042$ respectively); and to PHA-IL4 ($r= -0.6$ $p=0.03$).

Patient age was correlated negatively to IDC IL12p70 in both treated and untreated patients ($r= -0.6$ $p=0.025$, and $r= -0.5$ $p=0.03$ respectively).

In treated patients, the TLT parameter was correlated positively to sCD30 levels ($r=0.6$ $p=0.021$) in IDC supernatants and negatively to: IL10 and IL12p40 levels ($r= -0.5$ $p=0.044$ and $r= -0.5$ $p=0.042$ respectively) in IDC supernatants; IL12p70 in IDC-LPS supernatants ($r= -0.5$ $p=0.05$); IL10 in IDC-IFNβ supernatants($r= -0.5$ $p=0.045$); IFNγ, IL10, and IL4 in PBMC-PHA supernatants ($r= -0.5$ $p=0.039$, $r= -0.6$ $p=0.010$ and $r= 0.5$ $p=0.05$ respectively). The PHA-IL2 and -IL12p40, levels were correlated positively to the TD parameter ($r=0.6$ $p=0,032$ and $r= -0.6$ $p=0.015$ respectively) and PHA-IFNγ and -IL6 to treatment dose ($r= -0.5$ $p=0.05$ and $r= -0.6$ $p=0.029$ respectively).

IDC sCD30 and TH1/TH2/TH3 Cytokine Network Interactions

Correlation Analyses

In treated patients, significant negative correlation was found between levels of: IDC sCD30 and IL10 ($r= -0.6$ $p=0.023$) and positive correlation between levels of IDC sBcl2 and IL12p70 ($r=0.6$ $p=0.03$). Additionally, IDC production of IL10 was correlated positively to PHA-IL2 and -IFNγ levels($r=0.6$ $p=0.01$ and $r=0.5$ $p=0.05$ respectively), IDC production of TGFβ, was correlated positively to PHA-IL4 and -IL6 levels($r=0.5$ $p=0.044$ and $r=0.5$ $p=0.05$ respectively), IDC production of sBcl2, was correlated positively to PHA-IL4, -IL12p40 and -IFNγ levels ($r=0.7$ $p=0.01$, $r=0.6$ $p=0.02$ and $r=0.6$ $p=0.03$ respectively) and IDC production of IL12p40 was correlated positively to PHA-IL6 levels ($r=0.6$ $p=0.01$).

In untreated patients, significant negative correlation was found between levels of: IDC IL10 and PHA-IFNγ and -IL6 ($r= -0.5$ $p=0.02$ and $r= -0.7$ $p=0.003$ respectively) and positive correlation between levels of IDC sBcl2 and PHA-TGFβ ($r=0.9$ $p=0.0022$). IDC IL12p40 levels were correlated positively to PHA-IL2 and -IL10 ($r=0.7$ $p=0.001$ and $r=0.6$ $p=0.02$ respectively).

Covariance Analyses

These results are detailed in Tables 3 and 4. We noted that an increase of sCD30 levels in treated patients coincided with an increase in the levels of: TGFβ and IL12p40 in IDC supernatants (while sBcl2, IL10 and IL12p70 levels fell); IL6, IL12p70 and IL12p40 in PHA supernatants (while IL10, TGFβ, IL2, IFNγ and IL4 levels fell). In untreated patients an increase of sCD30 levels coincided with an increase in the levels of: IL12p70 and sBcl2 in IDC supernatants (while TGFβ, IL10 and IL12p40 levels fell); IL10, IL12p40, IL12p70 and IL4 in PHA supernatant (while TGFβ, IL6, IL2 and IFNγ levels fell).

Table 1. Treated and untreated patients: cytokine levels in DC culture supernatants

Cytokines	Levels of supernatant cytokines (pg/ml, °U/ml)												
	Untreated patients												
	n°	IDC			IDC–LPS			IDC–IFNβ			IDC–IFNγ		
IL10	18	3.0		0.8^{D}	*30.4		251.2^{D}	*0.8		2.2^{b}	3.7		1.0
IL12p70	18	*2.2		0.9^{a}	*4.4		25.5	3.3		0.6^{c}	*5.5		1.3^{d}
IL12p40	18	35.4		10.1^{E}	2028.0		438.6^{E}	*12.3		4.7	*10.3		178.2
TGFβ	18	3172.0		759.1	2922.2		720.1	2561.1		558.1	3115.7		684.0
°sCD30	18	*13.3		7.5^{e}	17.7		3.0^{f}	*10.9		4.7	19.0		3.0
°sBcl2	18	12.2		5.4	14.6		3.8	16.2		7.1	6.2		0.1
Treated patients													
	n°	IDC			IDC–LPS			IDC–IFNβ			IDC–IFNγ		
IL10	16	4.5		0.6^{A}	*7.2		434.9^{A}	*5.0		4.4^{b}	5.1		0.9
IL12p70	16	*0.8		0.2^{aB}	6.0		1.8^{B}	*1.4		0.6^{c}	*1.0		0.5^{d}
IL12p40	16	*15.3		18.1^{C}	826.4		447.0^{C}	*13.2		212.7	*45.5		47.2
TGFβ	16	3818.4		547.9	3229.8		601.2	3286.7		573.0	3267.9		549.8

Cytokine values are expressed as mean (or *median) ± standard error as appropriate.
Statistical differences between the groups were determined using the most appropriate statistical test depending on the population distribution :
^{aa} p= 0.014; ^{bb} p=0.045; ^{cc} p=0.047; ^{dd} p=0.0001; ^{ee} p=0.01; ^{ff} p=0.003
Statistical differences within groups were determined using ^Wilcoxon rank test for paired samples
^{AA} p=0.005; ^{BB} p=0.001; ^{CC} p=0.0007; ^{DD} p=0.005; ^{EE} p=0.0003; ^{FF} p=0.007;
^{GG} p=0.001; ^{HH} p=0.004; ^{II} p=0.009; ^{LL} p=0.01

Table 2. Whole blood

Cytokines	Levels of supernatant cytokines (pg/ml)							
	Untreated patients							
	n°	PBMC			PBMC–PHA			^1(p)
IL10	18	*1.8		0.2	*72.2		21.2	0.0003
IFNγ	13	18.1		2.7	2391.8		552.7 [b]	0.0004
IL6	18	*18.2		12.6	724.9		99.9	0.0004
IL2	18	*9.5		1.7	22.2		4.2	0.0004
IL4	18	0.6		0.1[a]	*1.6		1.2	0.0007
IL12p70	18	9.9		0.7	8.9		0.8	NS
IL12p40	18	21.1		4.3	*109.0		35.1	0.0006
TGFβ	18	*5094.0		3517.0	*8458.0		4627.0	NS
	Treated patients							
	n°	PBMC			PBMC–PHA			^1(p)
IL10	16	*1.8		0.2	22.3		11.8	0.0004
IFNγ	16	*14.2		3.3	684.3		152.1 [b]	0.0005
IL6	16	*9.3		42.8	796.4		112.6	0.0004
IL2	16	9.2		0.9	*13.5		7.9	0.0008
IL4	16	1.1		0.1 [a]	*3.6		1.2	0.006
IL12p70	16	8.7		0.6	10.3		0.8	NS
IL12p40	16	22.5		2.7	*103.5		22.2	0.0004
TGFβ	16	6229.7		505.1	7157.7		621.1	0.025

The cytokine values are expressed as mean (or *median) ± standard error as appropriate.
Statistical differences between the groups were determined using the most appropriate statistical test depending on the population distribution
[aa] p=0.007; [bb] p=0.007
Statistical differences within groups (^1 basic compared to PHA conditions) were determined using ^ Wilcoxon rank test for paired samples.

Table 3. Covariance between sCD30 and cytokine levels within the TH1/TH2/TH3 cytokine network

Untreated patients							
Increase of sCD30 in culture supernatants of:							
IDC		IDC + LPS (DC)		IDC + IFNβ (DC)		IDC + IFNγ (DC)	
↑ sBcl2	**↓ TGFβ**	**↑ sBcl2**	**↓ TGFβ**	**↑ IL10**	**↓ sBcl2**	**↑ sBcl2**	**↓ TGFβ**
↑ IL12p70	**↓ IL10**	*↑ IL12p40*	**↓ IL10**	**↑ IL12p70**	**↓ IL12p40**	*↑ IL12p70*	**↓ IL10**
↑ IL10	**↓ IL12p40**	*↑ IL4*	**↓ IL12p70**	*↑ TGFβ*	**↓ TGFβ**		**↓ IL12p70**
↑ IL12p40	*↓ TGFβ*	*↑ IL12p70*	**↓ IL12p40**	*↑ IL12p40*	*↓ IL10*		**↓ IL12p40**
↑ IL12p70	*↓ IL6*		*↓ TGFβ*	*↑ IL6*	*↓ IL4*		*↓ IL10*
↑ IL4	*↓ IL2*		*↓ IL2*	*↑ IL12p70*	*↓ IFNγ*		*↓ L12p40*
	↓ IFNγ		*↓ IL6*		*↓ IL2*		*↓ IL4*
			↓ IL10				*↓ IFNγ*
			↓ IFNγ				*↓ IL6*
							↓ IL2
							↓ TGFβ
Treated patients							
Increase of sCD30 in culture supernatants of:							
IDC		IDC + LPS (DC)		IDC + IFNβ (DC)		IDC + IFNγ (DC)	
↑ TGFβ	**↓ sBcl2**	**↑ TGFβ**	**↓ sBcl2**	**↑ sBcl2**	**↓ IL10**	**↑ TGFβ**	**↓ sBcl2**
↑ IL12p40	**↓ IL10**	**↑ IL10**	*↓ IL10*	**↑ IL12p70**	*↓ IL10*	**↑ IL12p70**	**↓ IL10**
↑ IL6	**↓ IL12p70**	**↑ IL12p70**	*↓ TGFβ*	**↑ IL12p40**	*↓ TGFβ*	**↑ IL12p40**	*↓ IL10*
↑ IL12p40	*↓ IL10*	**↑ IL12p40**	*↓ IL2*	**↑ TGFβ**	*↓ IL2*	*↑ IL4*	*↓ IL12p40*
↑ IL12p70	*↓ TGFβ*	*↑ IL6*	*↓ IL4*	*↑ IL6*	*↓ IFNγ*	*↑ IL6*	*↓ IL2*
	↓ IL2	*↑ IL12p40*	*↓ IFNγ*	*↑ IL4*		*↑ IL12p70*	
	↓ IFNγ	*↑ IL12p70*		*↑ IL12p40*		*↑ TGFβ*	
	↓ IL4			*↑ IL12p70*			

Covariance analyses between the level of sCD30 and cytokine production under the varying conditions:
↑ increase of production, ↓ decrease of production; **IDC, DC supernatants;** *Whole Blood supernatants*

Table 4. Covariance analyses in: 1:IDC supernatants; 2:IDC + LPS activation; 3:IDC+IFNβ activation; 4:IDC + IFNγ activation

Untreated patients																								
	sCD30				**sBcl2**				**IL10**				**IL12p70**				**IL12p40**				**TGFβ**			
	1	**2**	**3**	**4**	**1**	**2**	**3**	**4**	**1**	**2**	**3**	**4**	**1**	**2**	**3**	**4**	**1**	**2**	**3**	**4**	**1**	**2**	**3**	**4**
sCD30					+	+	-	+	-	-	+	-	+	-	+	-	-	-	-	-	-	-	-	-
sBcl2	+	+	-	+					+	-	-	+	-	+	-	-	-	-	-	-	-	-	-	+
IL10	-	-	+	-	+	-	-	+					+	+	-	-	+	+	-	+	+	+	+	+
IL12p70	+	-	+	-	-	+	-	-	+	+	-	-					-	+	-	+	-	+	-	-
IL12p40	-	-	-	-	-	-	-	-	+	+	-	+	-	+	-	+					+	+	+	+
TGFβ	-	-	-	-	-	-	-	+	+	+	+	+	-	+	-	-	+	+	+	+				
IL10	+	-	-	-	-	-	+	-	-	+	+	+	-	+	-	-	+	+	+	+	+	+	+	+
IFNγ	-	-	-	-	+	-	+	-	-	+	-	-	-	+	-	+	+	+	-	+	-	-	-	+
IL6	-	-	+	-	-	+	-	+	-	-	-	-	+	-	+	-	-	+	-	-	-	-	-	-
IL2	-	-	-	-	+	-	+	-	+	+	+	+	-	+	-	-	+	+	+	+	+	+	+	+
IL4	+	+	-	-	+	-	+	-	-	+	+	+	-	+	-	+	+	+	-	+	-	+	+	+
IL12p70	+	+	+	+	-	+	-	+	-	+	+	+	+	+	-	-	-	+	-	-	-	-	-	+
IL12p40	+	+	+	-	+	+	+	-	-	-	+	+	+	+	+	+	-	+	-	-	-	-	-	-
TGFβ	-	-	+	-	+	+	+	-	+	-	+	+	+	-	+	-	+	-	+	-	+	-	-	+
EDSS	-	+	+	+	-	-	-	+	-	+	-	-	+	-	+	-	-	-	-	-	-	-	-	-
Age	+	-	-	+	+	+	+	-	-	+	+	+	-	+	-	-	+	+	+	+	+	+	+	+
Treated patients																								
	sCD30				**sBcl2**				**IL10**				**IL12p70**				**IL12p40**				**TGFβ**			
	1	**2**	**3**	**4**	**1**	**2**	**3**	**4**	**1**	**2**	**3**	**4**	**1**	**2**	**3**	**4**	**1**	**2**	**3**	**4**	**1**	**2**	**3**	**4**
SCD30					-	-	+	-	-	+	-	-	-	+	+	+	+	+	+	+	+	+	+	+
SBcl2	-	-	+	-					+	+	-	-	+	-	+	+	+	-	-	-	+	-	+	-
IL10	-	+	-	-	+	+	-	-					-	+	+	-	-	+	+	+	-	+	+	-
IL12p70	-	+	+	+	+	-	+	+	-	+	+	-					+	+	+	+	+	+	+	+
IL12p40	+	+	+	+	+	-	-	-	-	+	+	+	+	+	+	+					+	+	+	+

Table 4. (Continued)

Treated patients																								
	sCD30				sBcl2				IL10				IL12p70				IL12p40				TGFβ			
	1	**2**	**3**	**4**	**1**	**2**	**3**	**4**	**1**	**2**	**3**	**4**	**1**	**2**	**3**	**4**	**1**	**2**	**3**	**4**	**1**	**2**	**3**	**4**
TGFβ	+	+	+	+	+	-	+	-	-	+	+	-	+	+	+	+	+	+	+	+				
IL10	-	-	-	-	+	-	+	-	+	+	+	+	-	+	-	-	+	+	+	+	-	+	+	+
IFNγ	-	-	-	-	+	+	+	+	+	-	+	+	-	-	-	-	+	+	+	+	-	+	-	-
IL6	+	+	+	+	+	+	+	-	-	+	-	-	+	+	+	+	+	+	-	+	+	+	+	+
IL2	-	-	-	-	+	+	-	-	+	+	+	+	+	+	+	-	-	+	+	-	-	-	-	-
IL4	-	-	+	+	+	+	-	-	+	-	+	+	-	-	-	-	+	-	+	+	+	+	+	-
IL12p70	+	+	+	+	+	-	+	-	+	+	+	+	-	+	+	-	+	-	+	+	+	+	+	+
IL12p40	+	+	+	-	+	+	+	-	+	+	+	+	-	+	-	-	+	+	-	+	+	+	+	+
TGFβ	-	-	-	+	+	-	-	-	+	-	+	+	+	+	-	-	-	-	+	-	+	+	+	+
EDSS	+	-	-	-	-	+	-	+	+	-	+	+	-	-	-	-	-	-	-	-	-	-	-	-
Age	+	-	+	-	-	+	+	+	+	-	+	+	-	-	-	-	+	-	-	+	+	-	-	-
TD	+	+	+	-	+	-	+	-	+	+	+	+	-	-	-	-	+	+	+	-	-	+	+	+
DOSE	+	-	+	-	-	+	-	-	-	+	-	-	+	+	+	+	-	-	-	-	-	-	--	
TLT	+	-	-	+	-	-	-	+	-	-	-	-	+	-	-	+	-	-	-	-	-	-	-	+

The covariance analyses produce a matrix of covariance coefficients between parameters, which can be positive or negative. Covariance measures the linear association between two parameters while controlling the possible effects of others. If both parameters increase or decrease at the same time, the covariance is positive whilst other changes are considered negative

Principal Component Analyses

By establishing the degree of correlation between parameters, these evaluations help clarify relationships by visualizing the functional-dynamics of the cellular network (F-dynamic-network). Confirming the correlation and covariance findings, the IDC F-dynamic-network (Fig.1) shows that: TH2 sp-IDC functions (IL10) (Fig.1a) oppose TH1-IDC functions (IL12p70) perfectly in treated patients, determining a balance between TH1 and TH2 IDC immunological functions (TH1/TH2). In untreated patients (Fig.1a), no balance exists between sp-IDC and TH1-IDC functions. Only type2 rIDC like immune response (rIDC2, TGFβ-IL12p40) functions were present in the F-dynamic-network of both treated and untreated patients. However, when the functional influence of sCD30 was evaluated (Fig.1b), we found that the balance between type 1 rIDC-like immune response (rIDC1, TGFβ-IL12p70) and rIDC2 was re-established in treated patients because of the fall in sCD30 levels (Table 1), due to the increase of sp-IDC (IL10) activity (sCD30 and sp-IDC vectors are perfectly opposed) and the consequent re-establishment of CD30-mediated signals. This would indicate that CD30 is involved in the physiological generation of rIDCs responsible for TH1/TH2/TH3 balance and that IDC CD30-mediated signals are absent in untreated patients. The importance of the rIDC1/rIDC2 balance emerges from the evaluation of the influence of F-dynamic-network on the EDSS parameter (Fig.1c): the balance between cells regulating type-1 (rIDC1) and type-2 (rIDC2) immune response opposes EDSS increase in treated patients, and rIDC2 function, when rIDC1 is lacking, determines TH1 disequilibrium (IL12p70↑) correlated to EDSS increase in untreated patients. The fall in sCD30 correlated to sp-DC activity is therefore an important immunological mechanism in the immune response and IFNβ–1a treatment. The F-dynamic-network between IDC and PHA-activated whole blood (WB) peripheral cells, considered T cells (Fig.1c), shows that: the balance between rIDC1/rIDC2 cells (TGFβ–IL12p70, -IL12p40) induces balance between peripheral Tr1s (WB TGFβ–IFNγ) and Tr2s (WB TGFβ–IL10), in treated patients (Fig.1c); while only rIDC2s (TGFβ–IL12p40) were present in the F-dynamic-network of untreated patients (as WB TGFβ does not interact with either WB IFNγ or IL10). The balance between rIDCs/Trs is dependent on the balance between rIDC1/rIDC2 precursor cells, as the sBcl2 IDC survival marker is interposed between WB IL12p70 and IL12p40, cytokines which regulate the macrophage type 1 or 2 IDC generation. In untreated patients, sBcl2 and sCD30 levels are positively correlated, clarifying the fact that an increase in sCD30 levels is linked to cell survival.

These findings demonstrate that: rIDCs, through CD30-mediated signals induce generation of Tr peripheral cells in treated patients, and that CD30 is involved in the cell contact-dependent suppression of TH cells by rIDCs, indispensable for the generation of TGFβ producing Trs (TH3 cells) involved in the control of TH1/TH2/TH3 balance of the immune response. In fact (Fig.1d): correlation exists between rIDC2s and rIDC1s (IDC TGFβ-IL12p40 and -IL12p70), and sCD30; Tr1s and Tr2s (WB TGFβ -IFNy and -IL10) were functionally present and also correlated. Additionally, the differing roles of IL4 and IL6 in the environment of the IDC F-dynamic-network was also highlighted: the former in the balance between macrophage type1/type2 generation (the WB IL4 vector was interposed between IL12p70 and IL12p40 vectors, which are the cytokines involved in the development of type1 and type2 macrophage cells respectively); the latter in IDC1/IDC2 balance (the WB IL6 vector was interposed between IDC IL12p70 and IL12p40 vectors). IL2 levels were correlated to sp-IDC function (IL10) confirming sp-DC activity as the main mechanism of suppression through IL2 activity [82].

Immature Dendritic Cells

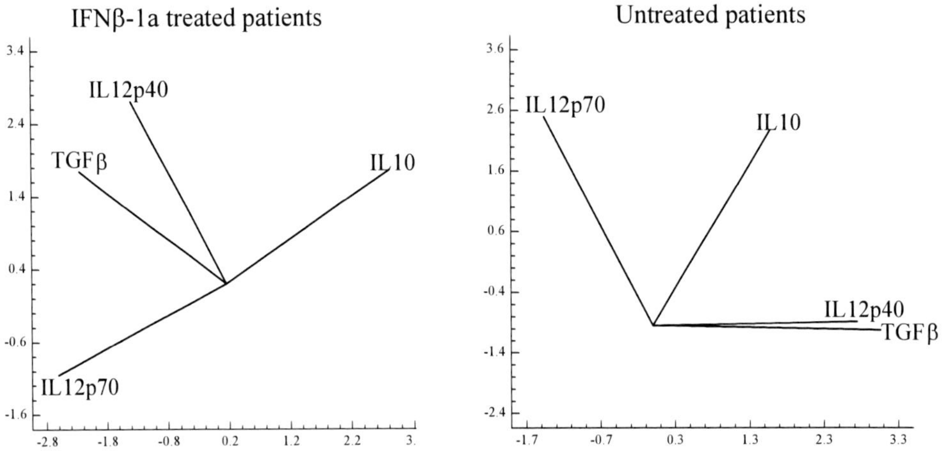

Figure 1a: Physiological conditions

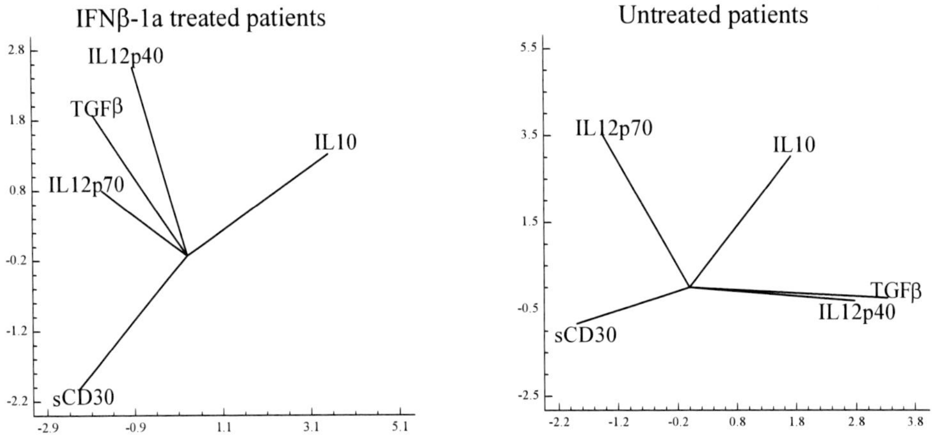

Figure 1b: Functional influence of sCD30 molecule

Figure 1. (Continues.)

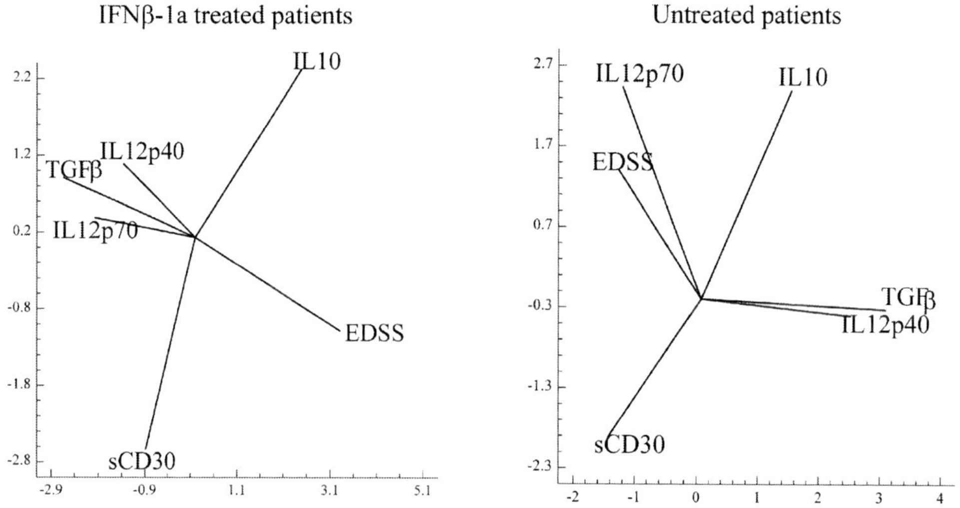

Figure 1c: Influence on EDSS parameter

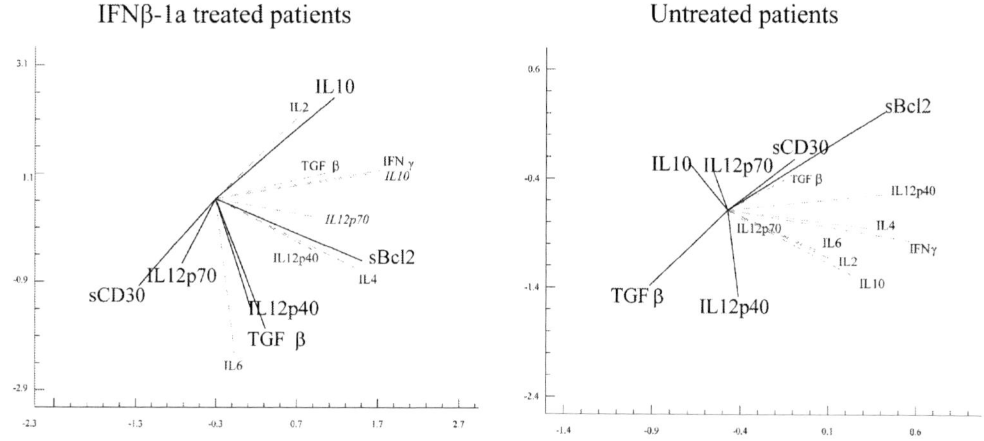

Figure 1d: Interactions between IDC and whole blood PHA activation (T cells)

Figure 1. Functional-dynamics of the cellular networks in treated and untreated patients: interactions between IDC TH1/TH2/TH3 immunological functions

IDC-LPS (DC) sCD30 and TH1/TH2 Cytokine Network Interactions

Correlation Analyses

In treated patients, significant positive correlation existed between: DC sCD30 and TGFβ (r=0.7 p=0.004), DC TGFβ and IL12p70 (r=0.5 p=0.05), DC IL12p70 and IL10 (r=0.7 p=0.004), IL10 and IL12p40 (r=0.5 p=0.032), DC IL12p70 and IL12p40 (r=0.8 p=0.004). In untreated patients, significant positive correlation was found between DC TGFβ and IL12p40 (r=0.5 p=0.036), DC IL10 and IL12p70 (r=0.7 p=0.003), and between DC IL12p70 and IL12p40 (r=0.5 p=0.048). Additionally, in treated patients, DC production of TGFβ was correlated positively to PHA-TGFβ, –IL4 and –IL6 levels(r=0.5 p=0.042, r=0.5 p=0.043 and r=0.7 p=0.005 respectively), and DC production of IL10 was correlated positively to PHA-IL2 levels (r=0.6 p=0.015).

In untreated patients DC production of TGFβ was positively correlated to PHA-IL2 (r=0.5 p=0.034), DC production of IL10 was positively correlated to PHA-IL10 and –IL2 (r=0.5 p=0.033 and r=0.7 p=0.003), DC production of IL12p70 was positively correlated to PHA-IL2 (r=0.6 p=0.014) and DC production of IL12p40 was positively correlated to PHA-IL2, -IFNγ and –IL10 (r=0.5 p=0.031, r=0.8 p=0.0003 and r=0.7 p=0.001 respectively).

Covariance Analyses

These results are detailed in Tables 3 and 4. An increase of sCD30 levels in treated patients was found to coincide with: an increase in the levels of TGFβ, IL10, IL12p70 and IL12p40 in the DC supernatants (while sBcl2 levels fell); an increase in the levels of IL6, IL12p70 and IL12p40 in the PHA supernatants (while IL10, TGFβ, IL2, IL4 and IFNγ levels fell). In untreated patients, an increase of sCD30 levels was found to coincide with: an increase in the levels of sBcl2 in the DC supernatants (while TGFβ, IL10, IL12p70 and IL12p40 levels fell); an increase in the levels of IL4, IL12p70 and IL12p40 in the PHA supernatants (while IL10, TGFβ, IL2, IL6 and IFNγ levels fell).

Principal Component Analyses

These analyses show that the fall in sCD30 levels in treated patients, highlighted by the study of statistical differences (Table 1), was determined by the increase in sp-DC activity (sp-DC and sCD30 vectors are opposed) (Fig.2b), thus re-establishing CD30-mediated signals and balance between rDC1 and rDC2 (TGFβ-IL12p70, -IL12p40 are positively correlated). This, in its turn, leads to balance between TH1/TH2/TH3 immune responses (Fig.2b). In untreated patients, sCD30 levels were higher and sp-DC activity did not determine a fall in sCD30 levels (Fig.2b) and hence CD30-mediated signals and the rDC1/rDC2 balance (TGFβ-IL12p70, -IL12p40 are not positively correlated), was not re-established, determining an imbalance (TH1↑) between TH1/TH2/TH3 immune responses (Fig.2a, 2b). In fact, when we evaluated the influence of the F-dynamic-network on EDSS increase we found that the TH1/TH2/TH3 balance (IL12p70/IL12p40/TGFβ) opposes EDSS increase (which was the outcome of the network) in the treated group (Fig.2c); whilst, the EDSS was the outcome between sp-DC activity and sCD30 increase in the untreated group (Fig.2c); only rDC2 functions were functionally present in the F-dynamic-network (Fig.2d). The evaluation of the F-dynamic-network of the interactions between DC and PHA-activated whole blood peripheral cells (T cells) (Fig.1c) showed a balance between rDC1/rDC2 cells in treated patients (DCIL12p70 and IL12p40 vectors were matched perfectly and were interposed between DC sCD30 and TGFβ vectors) and a balance between Tr1-Tr2 peripheral cells (the WB TGFβ was interposed between IFNγ and IL10 Fig.1c). While only rDC2 and Tr2 functions were present in the F-dynamic-network of untreated patients (Fig.2c). In treated patients (Fig.2d), sp-DC activity was closely correlated to rDC1/rDC2 balance, supporting its role in the re-establishment of this balance. Additionally, DC sBcl2 and sCD30 were negatively correlated in treated patients indicating that in the activated immune response, rDC CD30-mediated signals are involved in a negative selection of Trs, as in the thymus process (thus supporting the involvement of CD30 molecule in the Tr cell-cell contact mediated suppression by rDCs). Whereas, sBcl2 and sCD30 were positively correlated in untreated patients, clarifying the higher values in sCD30 levels of untreated patients and MS pathological mechanisms.

Immature Dendritic Cells + LPS *in vitro* stimulus

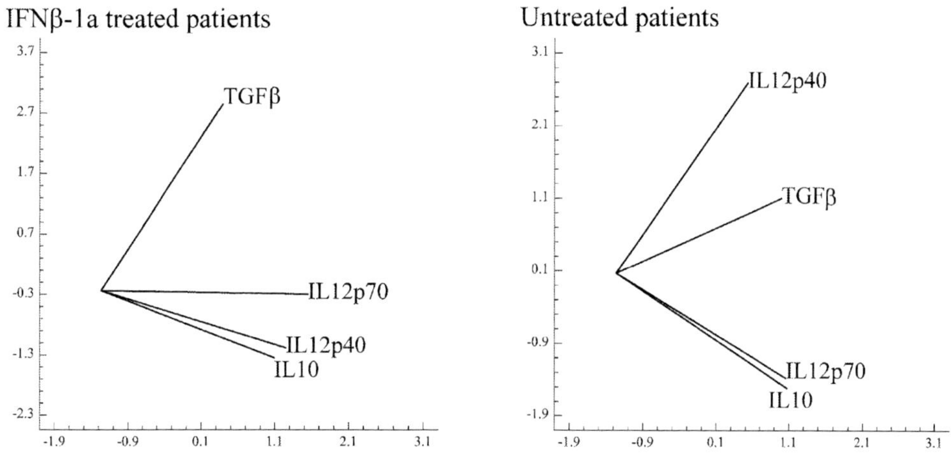

Figure 2a: Physiological conditions

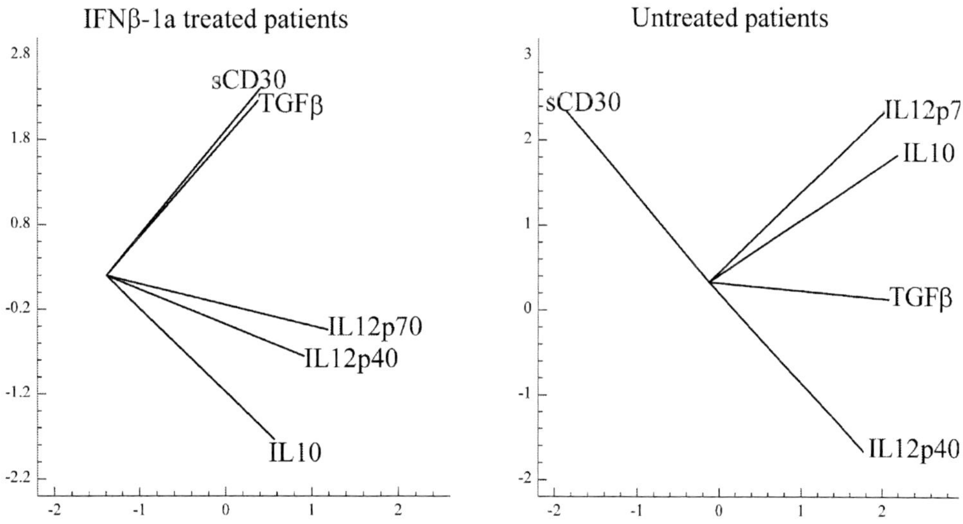

Figure 2b: Functional influence of sCD30 molecule

Figure 2. (Continues.)

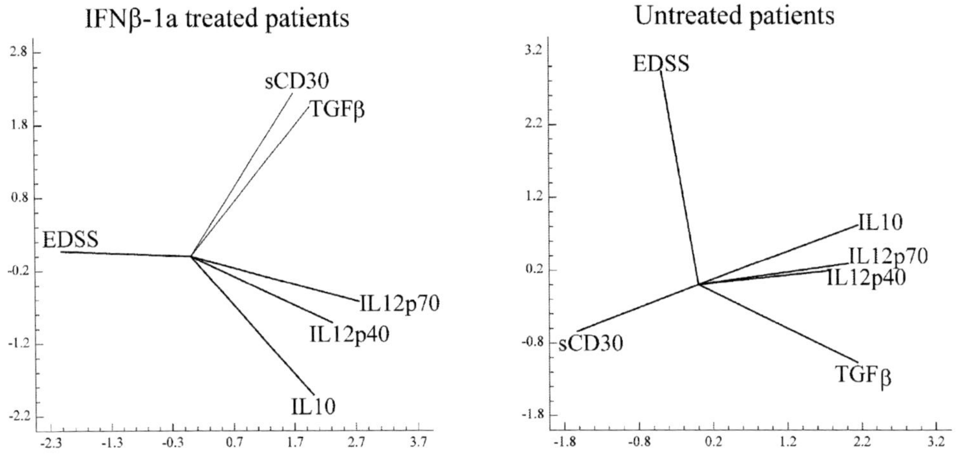

Figure 2c: Influence on EDSS parameter

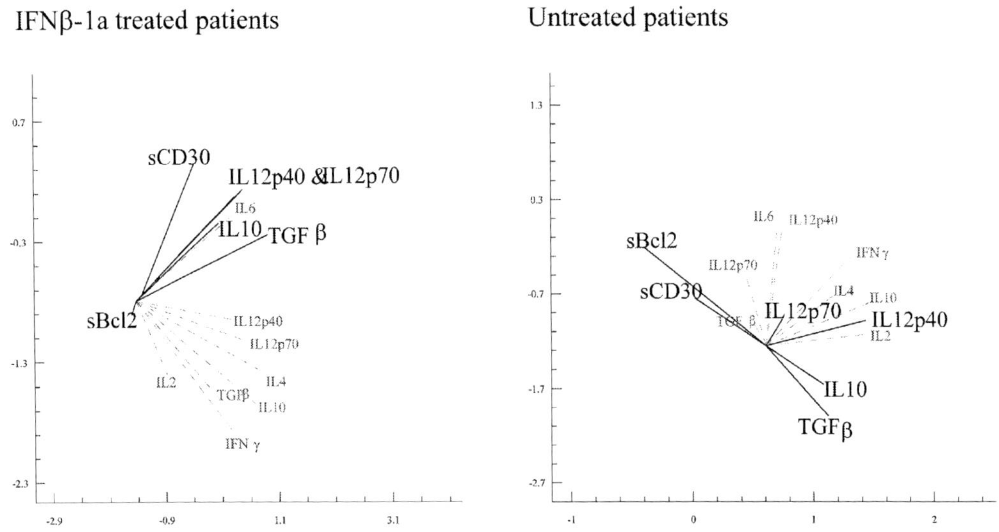

Figure 2d: Interactions between DC and whole blood PHA activation (T cells)

Figure 2. Functional-dynamics of the cellular networks in treated and untreated patients: interactions between DC (IDC + LPS stimulus) TH1/TH2/TH3 immunological functions

IDC-IFNβ (DC) sCD30 and TH1/TH2 Cytokine Network Interactions

Correlation Analyses

In treated patients, the correlation study revealed significant positive correlation between levels of DC sCD30 and TGFβ (r=0.6 p=0.002). Additionally, positive correlation was found between levels of: DC TGFβ and PHA-TGFβ and -IL6 (r=0.5 p=0.05 and r=0.6 p=0.006 respectively); DC Bcl2 and PHA-IL6 (r=0.6 p=0.02); DC IL10 and PHA-IL12p70 and –IL2 (r=0.5 p=0.03 and r=0.5 p=0.035 respectively); DC IL12p40 and PHA-IL12p70 (r=0.5 p=0.049). In untreated patients, positive correlations were found between levels of DC sCD30 and IL12p70 (rDC1, r=0.5 p=0.030), and negative between DC TGFβ and IL12p70 (r= –0.5 p=0.033). Furthermore, DC production of sBcl2 was positively correlated to PHA-TGFβ (r=0.9 p=0.007), DC production of IL10 was negatively correlated to PHA-IL6 (r= –0.5 p=0.044), DC production of IL12p70 was negatively correlated to PHA-IL10 (r= –0.5 p=0.024) and DC production of IL12p40 was positively correlated to PHA-IL2 (r=0.6 p=0.02).

Covariance Analyses

These results are shown in Tables 3 and 4. In treated patients an increase of DC sCD30 levels coincided with an increase in the levels of TGFβ, sBcl2, IL12p70 and IL12p40 (while IL10 levels fell) and an increase in the levels of PHA-IL4, -IL12p40, -IL6 and -IL12p70 (while PHA-IL10, -TGFβ, -IFNγ and -IL2 levels fell). In untreated patients, an increase of DC sCD30 levels coincided with an increase in the levels of IL10 and IL12p70 (while TGFβ, sBcl2, and IL12p40 levels fell) and an increase in the levels of PHA-TGFβ, -IL12p40, -IL6 and -IL12p70 (while PHA-IL10, -IL4, -IFNγ and -IL2 levels fell).

Principal Component Analyses

These results show how IFNβ *in vitro* alters patient immune responses according to whether they are receiving IFNβ–1a treatment or not. In fact, as the study of statistical differences showed (Table 1) (Fig.3) IFNβ induces a fall in sCD30 levels, in treated patients, by increasing sp-DC functional activity (IL10), determining a re-establishment of CD30-mediated signals and rDC1/rDC2 balance (TGFβ–IL12p70, -IL12p40) and hence balance between TH1/TH2/TH3 immune responses (TGFβ, IL12p70 and IL12p40 vectors were positively correlated) (Fig.3a, 3b). In untreated patients, there is no increase in sp-DC activity or decrease in sCD30 levels and consequently CD30-mediated signals and the balance between rDC1s/rDC2s are not re-established, determining an imbalance in TH1/TH2/TH3 immune responses (TGFβ, IL12p70 and IL12p40 vectors were negatively correlated) (Fig.2a, 2b). In fact, when we evaluated the influence of the F-dynamic-network on EDSS increase we found that (Fig.3c) TH1/TH2/TH3 balance (IL12p70/IL12p40/TGFβ) in the treated group opposed EDSS increase, sp-DC (IL10) opposed sCD30 increase and EDSS was the outcome of the network. In the untreated group, on the other hand, there was no balance between TH1/TH2/TH3 functions, sp-DC (IL10) did not oppose sCD30 increase and the EDSS was the outcome of sCD30 and TH1 function increase (IL12p70 cytokine) (Fig.3c)

The evaluation of the F-dynamic-network interactions between DC and PHA-activated whole blood peripheral cells (T cells) (Fig.3d) showed balance between rDC1/rDC2 cells and between Tr1/Tr2 peripheral cells, in treated patients (Fig.3c); while only Dr2 and Tr1 functions were present in the F-dynamic-network of untreated patients (Fig.3c). Interestingly, the balance between rDC1/rDC2 and Tr1/Tr2 is obtained by an initial generation of rDC1s and Tr1s, and a subsequent development of rDC2s and Tr2s (Fig.3d): precursor rDC1s

(TGFβ–IL12p70) are correlated to rDC2s (WB IL4–IL12p40 which are the cytokines involved in the rDC2 development from type 2 macrophage cells); Tr1 cells (WB TGFβ–IFNγ) are correlated to Tr2 development (because WB TGFβ–IFNγ was correlated to IL10); rDC2 induction is regulated by the TH1 T cell function (DC-IL12p40 is closely correlated positively to WB IFNγ).

Immature Dendritic Cells + IFNβ *in vitro* stimulus

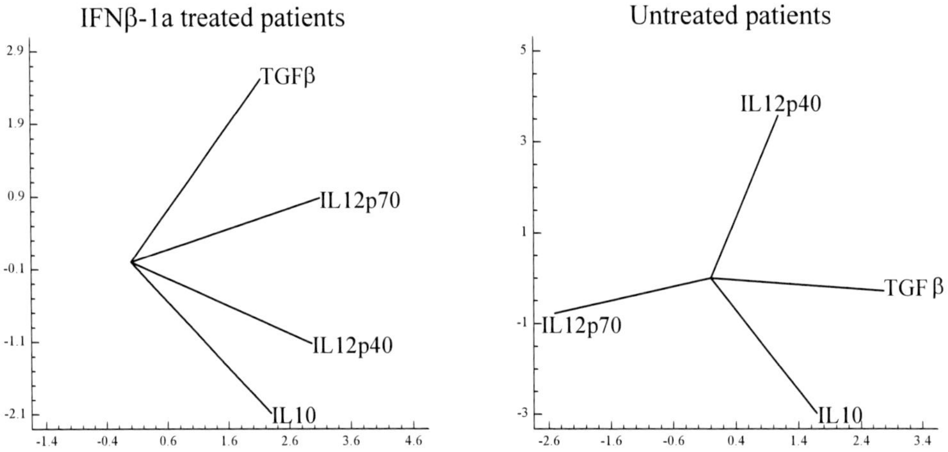

Figure 3a: Physiological conditions

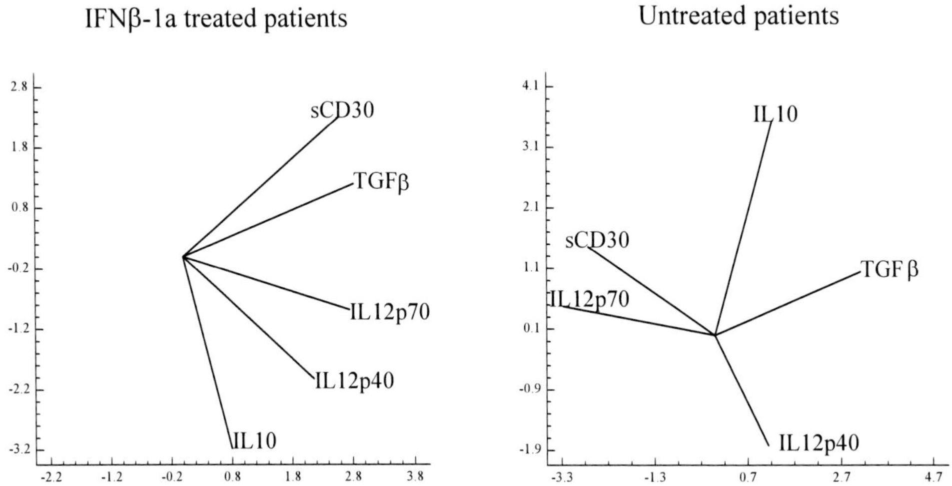

Figure 3b: Functional influence of sCD30 molecule

Figure 3. (Continues.)

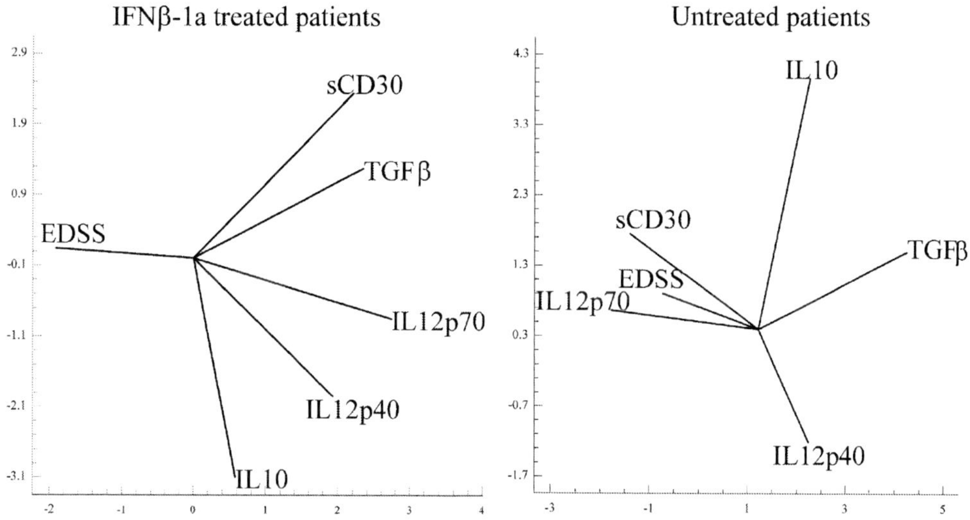

Figure 3c: Influence on EDSS parameter

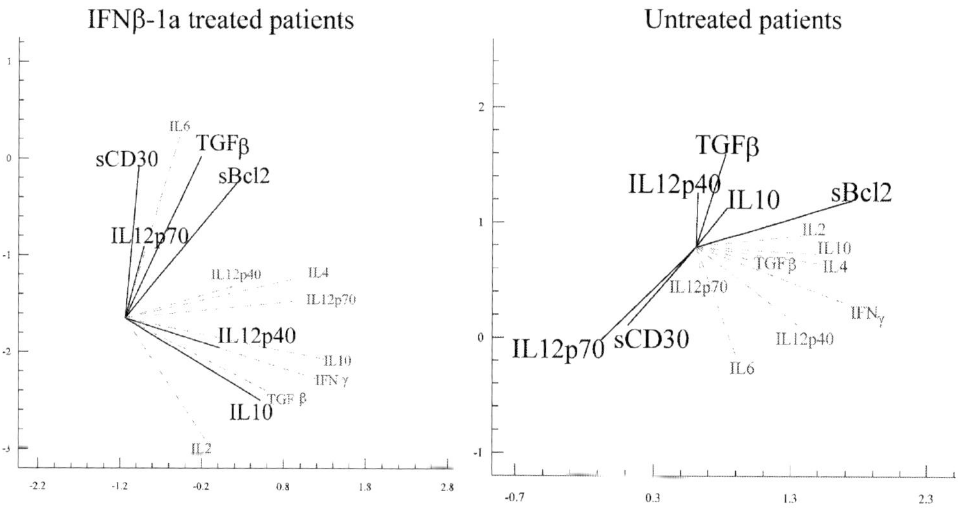

Figure 3d: Interactions between DC and whole blood PHA activation (T cells)

Figure 3. Functional-dynamics of the cellular networks in treated and untreated patients: interactions between DC (IDC + IFNβ stimulus) TH1/TH2/TH3 immunological functions

IDC-IFNγ (DC) sCD30 and TH1/TH2/TH3 Cytokine Network Interactions

Correlation Analyses

In treated patients, the level of DC sCD30 was correlated negatively to IL10 ($r= -0.5$ $p=0.026$) and positively to TGFβ ($r=0.7$ $p=0.04$). Additionally, positive correlation was found between levels of: DC TGFβ and PHA-TGFβ, -IL12p70 and -IL6 ($r=0.7$ $p=0.008$, r=0.5 p=0.048 and r=0.6 p=0.019 respectively); and negative correlation between levels of DC IL12p70 and PHA-IFNγ (r= –0.6 p=0.018). In untreated patients, an increase of DC TGFβ was positively correlated to IL12p40 (r=0.6 p=0.02), an increase of DC sCD30 was negatively correlated to PHA-TGFβ (r= –0.5 p=0.05), an increase of DC IL10 was positively correlated to PHA-IL2 and -IL10 (r=0.5 p=0.03 and r=0.5 p=0.048 respectively), and an increase of DC IL12p40 was positively correlated to PHA-IL2 (r=0.6 p=0.009).

Covariance Analyses

These results are shown in Tables 3 and 4. In treated patients, an increase of DC sCD30 levels coincided with an increase in the levels of TGFβ, L12p70 and IL12p40 (while sBcl2 and IL10 fell) and an increase in the levels of PHA-TGFβ, -IL4, -IL6 and -IL12p70 (while PHA-IL10, -IL12p40 and -IFNγ levels fell).

In untreated patients, an increase of DC sCD30 levels coincided with an increase in sBcl2 levels (while IL10, IL12p70 and IL12p40 levels fell) and an increase in the levels of PHA-IL12p70 (while PHA-TGFβ, -IL4, -IL6, -IL10, -IL12p40 and -IFNγ levels fell).

Principal Component Analyses

The results of the DC F-dynamic-network in IFNγ *in vitro* conditions show how IFNγ stimulus influences immune response in treated and untreated MS patients differently. In treated patients, (Fig.4), IFNγ stimulus induces an increase of sp-DC (IL10) activity determining a fall in TH1 (IL12p70) activity, while sCD30 was involved in the generation of rDC2 (TGFβ-IL12p40) cells, which maintain the balance between TH1/TH2 (IL12p70/IL10) immune responses (Fig.4a, 4b). In untreated patients, rDC2 TGFβ-IL12p40) cells were functionally present in the DC F-dynamic-network in IFNγ conditions but IFNγ stimulus did not determine an increase in sp-DC activity (IL10) or a fall in sCD30 levels and consequently CD30-mediated signals were not re-established. In fact, when we evaluated the influence of F-dynamic-network on EDSS increase (Fig.4c) we found that EDSS increase was opposed by the TH1/TH2 (IL12p70/IL12p40) balance in the treated group and that this function was regulated by CD30 regulatory cells (TGFβ-sCD30) and that sp-DC (IL10) increase opposed CD30 increase. In the untreated group, rDC2s (TGFβ-IL12p40) were functionally present but sp-DC activity did not oppose sCD30 increase and there was no balance between TH1/TH2/TH3 functions in opposition to the EDSS increase, which was correlated to sCD30 increase (Fig.4c).

The evaluation of the F-dynamic-network interactions between DC and PHA-activated whole blood peripheral cells (T cells) (Fig.4d) showed that there was a balance between rDC1/rDC2 cells and between Tr1/Tr2 peripheral cells, in treated patients. This balance did not exist in untreated patients (neither rDC1s/rDC2s nor Tr1s/Tr2s were present).

Comparing IFNβ and IFNγ stimulated (*in vitro)* F-dynamic- networks of treated patients (Fig.3d and 4d respectively), the functional interactions between DC and T cells demonstrate that CD30 mediated signals regulate physiological mechanisms of key importance for the balance between TH1/TH2/TH3 functions. In fact, the presence of IFNγ stimulus also determined balance between rDC1s/rDC2s and Tr1s/Tr2s, but through an opposing mechanism with respect to the IFNβ stimulus: rDC2s (DC TGFβ-IL12p40) and Tr2s (WB TGFβ-IL4) were generated first, but the increase of the former cells is correlated to an increase of precursor rDC1s (IL4 and IL12p70, which are cytokines involved in the development of rDC1s from type 1 macrophage cells), whilst the increase of the latter cells was correlated to the increase of Tr1s (WB TGFβ-IL4, -IL10 and -IFNγ were correlated); this balance was regulated by TH1-DC functions (WB TGFβ-IL4, -IL10 and -IFNγ were negatively correlated to DC-IL12p70)

Immature Dendritic Cells + IFNγ *in vitro* stimulus

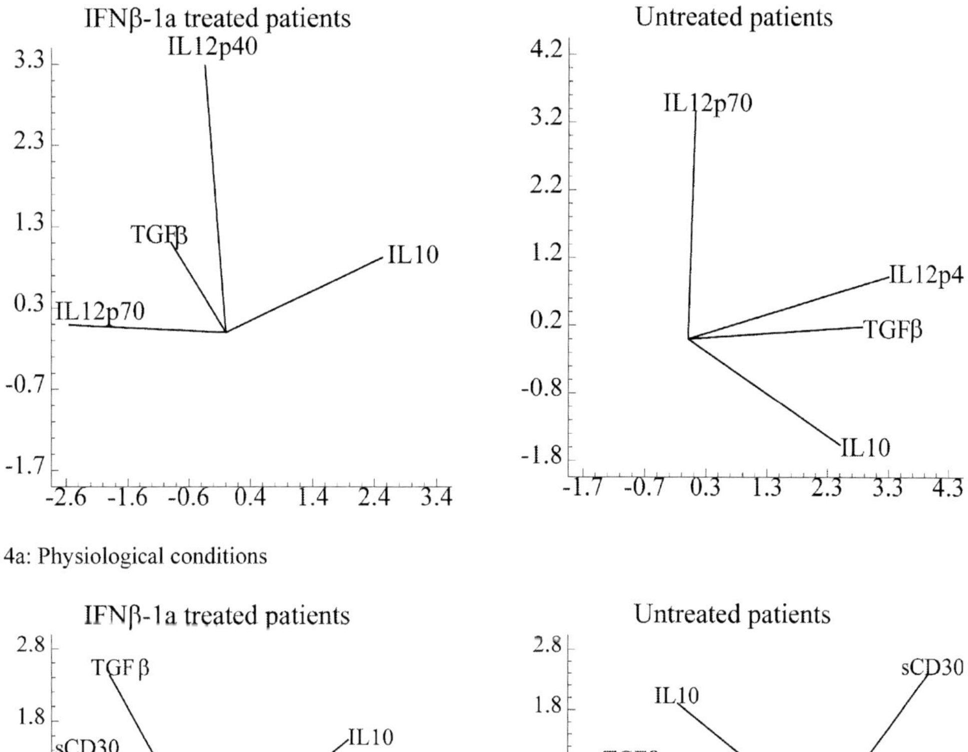

Figure 4a: Physiological conditions

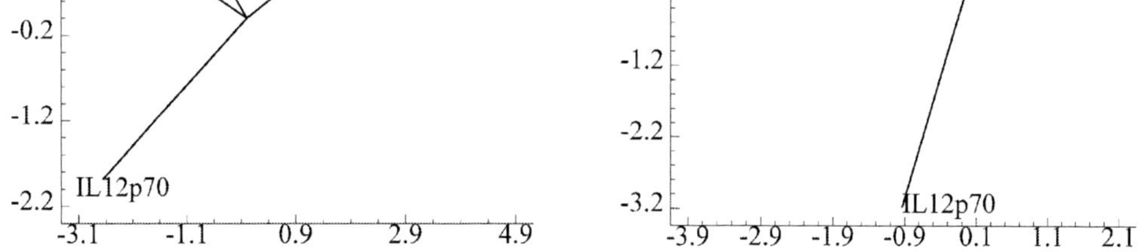

Figure 4b: Functional influence of sCD30 molecule

Figure 4. (Continues.)

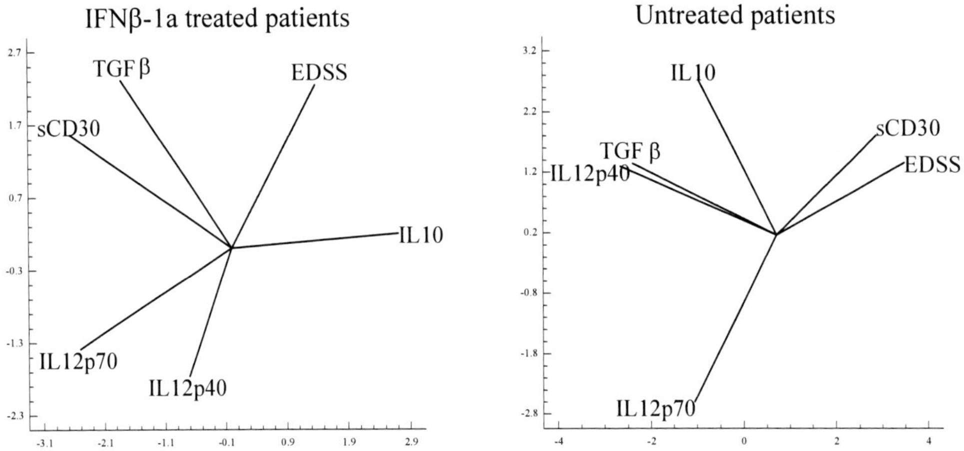

Figure 4c: Influence on EDSS parameter

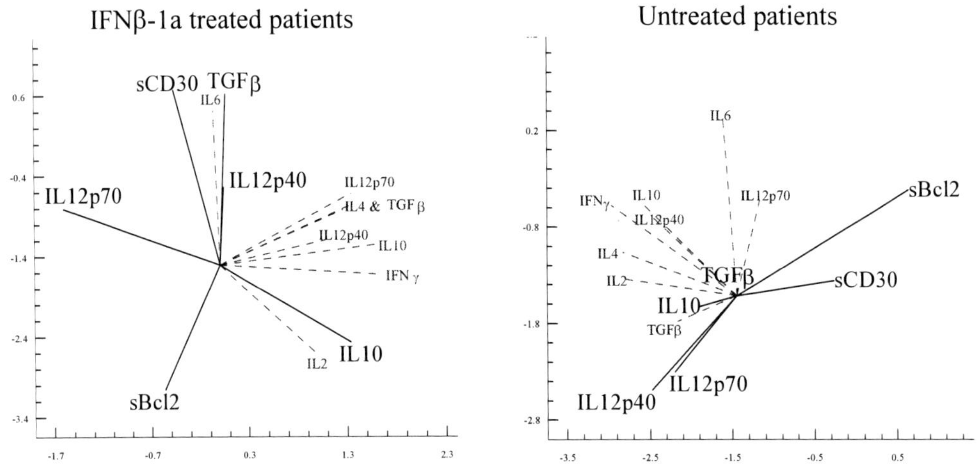

Figure 4d: Interactions between DC and whole blood PHA activation (T cells)

Figure 4. Functional-dynamics of the cellular networks in treated and untreated patients: interactions between DC (IDC + IFNγ stimulus) TH1/TH2/TH3 immunological functions

Conclusion

Our overall results indicate that the CD30 molecule is involved in the physiological generation and balance of rIDC1s/rIDC2s and rDC1s/rDC2s subsets of IDCs and DCs, in resting and activated immune response conditions. Our data also indicate that CD30 is involved in the cell contact-dependent suppression between rIDCs, rDCs and TH cells, indispensable for the generation of Tr1- and Tr2- TGFβ producing (TH3) subsets involved in maintaining the balance between TH1/TH2/TH3 type immune responses and central and peripheral immune tolerance. Alterations in these immunological mechanisms were found in untreated patients, while IFNβ–1a treatment was found to partially restore physiological mechanisms.

These conclusions are drawn from our results showing that an abnormal increase in sCD30 levels in untreated patients (Table 1) produces a disruption in: the generation and balance between rIDC1/rIDC2 and rDC1/rDC2 subsets; rIDCs/rDCs induction and balance of the Tr1 and Tr2 subsets and consequently, the balance between TH1/TH2/TH3 immune responses (Fig.1-4).

In treated patients, IFNβ–1a treatment was found to induce an increase in the activity of sp-IDC and sp-DC activity (IL10 cytokine), in resting and activated immune conditions (LPS) determining a fall in sCD30 levels, thus re-establishing CD30-mediated signals and the functional balance between rIDC1s, rDC1s (TGFβ-IL12p70) and rIDC2s, rDC2s (TGFβ–IL12p40). This in its turn, through the costimulator molecule CD30, induces the generation and balance between Tr1s (TGFβ-IFNγ) and Tr2s (TGFβ-IL10 and -IL4), re-establishing balance between TH1/TH2/TH3 immune responses and central and peripheral tolerance (Fig.1-4). However, we also noted that although rIDCs and rDCs are able to induce normal control in resting (IDC) and activated (DC) TH1/TH2/TH3 immune responses *in vitro*, this was only partial *in vivo*, as indicated by the EDSS parameter: positive correlation between the increases in EDSS and a fall in rDC1 activity (TGFβ-IL12p70) in immune activation conditions (LPS) in treated patients, despite rDC, Tr and TH1/TH2/TH3 network balance found *in vitro* (DC-LPS supernatants). We believe that rDC1 immune functions are suppressed *in vivo*, as a result of IFNβ–1a treatment itself and that this suppression is probably why IFNβ–1a treatment fails to resolve the disease completely: rDC1 immune functions (TGFβ-IL12p70) are normally involved *in vivo* mechanisms leading to the elimination of self-reactive cells. In fact, in experimental research into autoimmunity [99,100] and encephalomyelitis [101], an animal model of MS, the mechanisms involved in the destruction of self-aggressive cells and prevention of relapse and EDSS were found to be mediated by DCs inducing TGFβ-IFNγ production, and IL12p70 is the principal IFNγ inducer.

Generally IFNβ, by phosphorylating signal transducers and activators of transcription (STAT)4 cytoplasmic proteins, promotes IFNγ production and induces TH1 immune response. However, IFNβ induction of STAT4 expression has been found to be regulated by environment TH2 cytokines [102] and IL10 was found to suppress the expression of STAT4 in DCs and macrophages when present during maturation and activation, resulting in a fall of IFNγ production. We, too, noted this fall linked to an increase of IL10 and IL4 cytokines (TH2↑) in treated patients and this lends weight to our theory that IFNβ–1a fails to resolve MS completely due to an *in vivo* suppression of rDC1 immune functions. In other words *in vivo*, IFNβ–1a treatment determines TH2↑ physiological conditions, which suppress the expression of STAT4 in DCs and macrophages during the maturation and activation immunological phases; this situation induces re-establishment of CD30-mediated-signals but not rDC1/Tr1 activity in activation conditions necessary for the destruction of self-aggressive cells.

When IFNβ was used as an *in vitro* stimulus, the immunological mechanisms behind IFNβ–1a treatment and its differing effects on patient immune responses, according to whether patients were receiving IFNβ–1a treatment or not, became clearer. In fact, significantly higher (↑) values of IL10 (sp-DC) were found in the IDC-IFNβ supernatants of treated patients, while levels of IL12p70 were higher (TH1↑) in the IDC, IDC-IFNβ and IDC-

IFNγ supernatants of untreated patients (Table 1). Additionally, in treated patients, the IDC and DC- F-dynamic network (Fig.3), in which physiological TH2↑ conditions had suppressed the expression of STAT4 IFNβ was found to induce a fall in sCD30 levels by increasing sp-DC functional activity (IL10), thus determining: a re-establishment of CD30-mediated signals, rDC1/rDC2, Tr1/Tr2 balance and balance between TH1/TH2/TH3 immune responses (Fig.3a, 3b). In untreated patients, on the other hand, IFNβ did not induce an increase in sp-DC activity or a decrease in sCD30 levels; CD30-mediated signals were not re-established and consequently neither the balance between rDC1s/rDC2s which determined an imbalance between TH1/TH2/TH3 immune responses (Fig.2a, 2b). When we evaluated the influence of the F-dynamic network on EDSS increase we found that TH1/TH2/TH3 balance (IL12p70/IL12p40/TGFβ) opposed EDSS increase, sp-DC (IL10) opposed sCD30 increase and EDSS was the outcome of the network, in the treated group (Fig.3c). In the untreated group, there was no balance between TH1/TH2/TH3 functions, sp-DC (IL10) did not oppose sCD30 increase and the EDSS was the outcome of sCD30 and TH1 function (IL12p70 cytokine) increase (Fig.3c). Using IFNβ as an *in vitro* stimulus (Fig.3d), there was a balance between rDC1s/rDC2s and between peripheral Tr1s/Tr2s, in treated patients (Fig.3d) while only Dr2 and Tr1 functions were present in the F-dynamic-network of untreated patients (Fig.1d).

Our results from IFNγ *in vitro* stimulus also shows how IFNγ stimulus influences the immune response of treated and untreated MS patients differently (Fig.4). In treated patients, IFNy stimulus induces an increase of sp-DC (IL10) activity determining a fall in TH1 (IL12p70) activity, while sCD30 was involved in the generation of rDC2s (TGFβ-IL12p40), which maintain the balance between TH1/TH2/TH3 (IL12p70/IL10/TGFβ) immune responses (Fig.4a, 4b). In untreated patients, rDC2s (TGFβ-IL12p40) were functionally present in the DC F-dynamic-network, but IFNγ stimulus did not determine an increase in sp-DC activity (IL10) or a decrease in sCD30 levels, and consequently there was no re-establishment of CD30-mediated signals. In the treated group (Fig.4c) EDSS increase is opposed by TH1-TH2 (IL12p70-IL12p40) balance and this function is regulated by CD30 regulatory cells (TGFβ-sCD30) whilst sp-DC (IL10) increase opposes CD30 increase. In the untreated group, rDC2s (TGFβ-IL12p40) are present but sp-DC activity does not oppose sCD30 increase and no balance exists between TH1/TH2/TH3 functions to oppose EDSS increase which is correlated to sCD30 increase (Fig.4c). The evaluation of the F-dynamic-network interactions between DC and PHA-activated whole blood peripheral cells (T cells) (Fig.4d) showed that there was a balance between rDC1s/rDC2s and between peripheral Tr1s/Tr2s, in treated patients while this balance did not exist in untreated patients.

Interestingly, the evaluations of the treated patient activated F-dynamic-networks, (Fig.1-4d), demonstrate that CD30-mediated signals regulate physiological mechanisms of key importance for the immunological homeostasis between TH1/TH2/TH3 functions and central and peripheral tolerance. In the case of an unspecific stimulus, such as LPS, a perfect functional balance existed between rDC1s/rDC2s and Tr1s-Tr2s. When IFNβ *in vitro* stimulus was used, the balance between rDC1s/rDC2s and Tr1s/Tr2 is obtained by an initial generation of rDC1s and Tr1s, and subsequent development of rDC2s and Tr2s (Fig.3d): precursor rDC1s (TGFβ-IL12p70) are correlated to rDC2s (WB IL4-IL12p40 which are the cytokines involved in the rDC2 development from type 2 macrophage cells); Tr1 cells (WB TGFβ-IFNγ) are correlated to Tr2 development (because WB TGFβ-IFNγ was correlated to

IL10); and rDC2 induction is regulated by TH1 T cell function (DC-IL12p40 is closely correlated positively to WB IFNγ).

The presence of IFNγ stimulus, on the other hand, determined balance between rDC1s/rDC2s and Tr1s/Tr2s, but through an opposing mechanism with respect to IFNβ stimulus: rDC2s (DC TGFβ-IL12p40) and Tr2s (WB TGFβ-IL4) were generated first, but the increase of the former cells was correlated to an increase of precursor rDC1s (IL4-IL12p70 which are cytokines involved in rDC1 development from type 1 macrophage cells), whilst the increase of the latter cells was correlated to an increase of Tr1s (WB TGFβ-IL4, -IL10 and -IFNγ were correlated); this balance was regulated by TH1-DC functions (WB TGFβ-IL4, -IL10 and -IFNγ were negatively correlated to DC-IL12p70)

The negative correlation between DC sBcl2 and sCD30 in treated patients indicates that rDC CD30-mediated signals are involved in a negative selection of Trs in the activated immune response, as in the thymus process, thus supporting the involvement of the CD30 molecule in the Tr-cell contact mediated suppression by rDCs. Whereas, the positive correlation between sBcl2 and sCD30 in untreated patients clarifies the higher sCD30 values and MS pathological mechanisms.

As mentioned earlier, another objective of this study was to identify methods for re-establishing the physiological function of regulatory cells in autoimmunity diseases, such as MS, and more effective strategies for the prevention and treatment of immunopathological conditions such as transplant rejection, allergy and tumor. Our data show that sCD30 and IL4, IL6 and IL2 cytokine levels have differing roles in the environment of the IDC F-dynamic-network (Fig1-4d). sCD30 is a marker for the normal functioning of CD30 molecule-mediated signals and, so, for the normal regulatory mechanisms involved in the balance between TH1/TH2/TH3 immune responses and central and peripheral tolerance; IL4 is involved in the balance between macrophage type1/type2 generation (WB IL4 vector was interposed between IL12p70 and IL12p40 vectors, which are the cytokines involved in the development of type1 and type2 macrophage cells respectively); whilst IL6, is involved in the IDC1/IDC2 balance (WB IL6 vector was interposed between IDC IL12p70 and IL12p40 vectors). It has been shown that IL6 switches the differentiation of monocytes from IDC to macrophage cells [103], and that IL4 antagonizes this action [104]. This inhibition was found to be correlated to IL6 environmental concentration, while the IL4 action was found to involve down regulation of the expression of macrophage-colony stimulatory factor receptors. Our results show that IL2 levels are correlated to sp-IDC function (IL10) confirming the sp-DC suppressive function through IL2 activity [82]. Therefore, the importance of sCD30, IL6, IL4 and IL2 levels as markers for the balance of the TH1/TH2/TH3 immune responses and, consequently, for the physiological homeostasis, is clear (as we previously showed [105,106]). Whilst the fact that IFNβ–1a treatment is only effective in a resting state of the immune system is an important consideration that needs to be taken into account for an effective DC-immunotherapy in MS patients. Our results suggest that the main cause of treatment failure is the suppression of regulatory rIDC/rDC/Tr functions within the physiological activity of the immune system in activation conditions.

Summing up our results indicate that the CD30 molecule is involved in the cell contact-dependent suppression of TH cells by rIDCs, and rDCs and that this contact-dependent suppression is indispensable for the generation of TGFβ producing Tr (TH3) subsets. Alterations at this level were found in untreated patients, while IFNβ–1a treatment was found to restore the physiological mechanisms in treated patients by increasing suppressive (sp-) IDC and sp-DC (IL10) activity, resulting in a lowering of sCD30 levels, re-establishment of CD30-mediated signals and equilibrium between rIDC1s/rIDC2s and rDC1s/rDC2s. Consequently, CD30 being responsible for the balance between Tr1/Tr2, re-establishes equilibrium between immune responses and central and peripheral tolerance. However it would also appear that IFNβ–1a treatment is responsible for the *in vivo* suppression of patient TH1-DC functions which are responsible for the induction of Tr1s for the deletion of self aggressive cells in the immune response in activation conditions.

We conclude that CD30 is responsible for the physiological mechanisms involved in and regulating the cell contact-dependent suppression of Trs by rIDCs/rDCs and consequently in the balance between resting/activated immune responses and central and peripheral tolerance. Therefore CD30 is an exclusive and specific costimulatory molecule, and marker for rIDC/rDC/Tr subpopulations for immunotherapy study, selection and treatment. Further study could lead the way to identifying methods for re-establishing the physiological function of regulatory cells in autoimmunity diseases, such as MS, and more effective strategies for the prevention and treatment of immunopathological conditions such as transplant rejection, allergy and tumor.

References

[1] Durkop, H; Latza, U; Hummel, M; Eitelbach, F; Seed, B; Stein H. Molecular cloning and expression of a new member of the nerve growth factor receptor family that is characteristic for Hodgkin's disease. *Cell*, 1992 68,421-427.

[2] Smith, CA; Gruss, HJ; Davis, T; Anderson, D; Farrah, T; Baker, E; Sutherland, GR; Brannan, CI; Copeland, NG; Jenkins, NA. CD30 antigen, a marker for Hodgkin's lymphoma, is a receptor whose ligand defines an emerging family of cytokines with homology to TNF. *Cell,* 1993 73,1349-1360.

[3] Smith, CA; Farrah, T; Goodwin, RG. The TNF receptor superfamily of cellular and viral proteins: activation, costimulation, and death. *Cell,* 1994 76,959-962.

[4] Schwab, U; Stein, H; Gerdes, J; Lemke, H; Kirchner, H; Schaadt, M; Diehl, V. Production of a monoclonal antibody specific for Hodking and Stemberg-Reed cell of Hodgkin's disease and a subset of normal lymphoid cells. *Nature,* 1982 299,65-67.

[5] Stein, H; Mason, DY; Gerdes, J; O'Connor, N; Wainscoat, J; Pallesen, G; Gatter, K; Falini, B; Delsol, G; Lemke, H. The expression of the Hodgkin's disease associated antigen Ki-1 in reactive and neoplastic lymphoid tissue: evidence that Reed-Sternberg cells and histiocytic malignancies are derived from activated lymphoid cells. *Blood,* 1985 66,848-858.

[6] Gruss, HJ; Dower, SK. Tumor necrosis factor ligand superfamily: involvement in the pathology of malignant lymphomas. *Blood,* 1995 85,3378-3404.

[7] Madsen, JC; Peugh, WN; Wood, KJ; Morris, PJ. The effect of anti-L3T4 monoclonal antibody treatment on first-set rejection of murine cardiac allografts. *Transplantation,* 1987 44,849-852.

[8] Alzona, M; Jack, HM; Fisher, RI; Ellis, TM. CD30 defines a subset of activated human T cells that produce IFN-gamma and IL-5 and exhibit enhanced B cell helper activity. *J Immunol,* 1994 153,2861-2867.

[9] Gerli, R; Lunardi, C; Vinante, F; Bistoni, O; Pizzolo, G; Pitzalis, C. Role of CD30+ T cells in rheumatoid arthritis: a counter-regulatory paradigm for Th1-driven diseases. *Trends in Immunology,* 2001 22, 72-76.

[10] Kadin, E M. Commentary: Regulation of CD30 antigen expression and its potential significance for human disease. *Am. J of Pathol,* 2002 156,14769-1484.

[11] Muta, H; Boise, LH; Fang, L; Podack, ER. CD30 signals integrate expression of cytotoxic effector molecules, lymphocyte trafficking signals, and signals for proliferation and apoptosis. *J Immunol,* 2000 165,5105-5111.

[12] Duckett, SC; Thompson, BC. CD30-dependent degradation of TRAF2:implications for negative regulation of TRAF signalling and the control of cell survival. *Genes & development,* 1997 11,2810-2821.

[13] Jumper, MD; Fujita, K; Lipsky, PE; Meek, K. A CD30 responsive element in the germline promoter that is distinct from and inhibitory to the CD40 response element. *Molecular Immunol,* 1996 33,965-972.

[14] McDonald, PP; Cassatella, MA; Bald, A; Maggi, E; Romagnani, S; Gruss, HJ; Pizzolo, G. CD30 ligation induces nuclear factor-kappa B activation in human T cell lines. *Eur J Immunol,* 1995 25,2870-2876.

[15] Ansieau, S; Scheffrahn, I; Mosialos, G; Brand, H; Duyster, J; Kaye, K; Harada, J; Dougall, B; Hubinger, G; Kieff, E; Herrmann, F; Leutz, A; Gruss, HJ. Tumor necrosis factor receptor-associated factor (TRAF)-1, TRAF-2, and TRAF-3 interact *in vivo* with the CD30 cytoplasmic domain; TRAF-2 mediates CD30-induced nuclear factor kappa B activation. *Proc Natl Acad Sci U S A,* 1996 93,14053-8.

[16] Aizawa, S; Nakano, H; Ishida, T; Horie, R; Nagai, M; Ito, K; Yagita, H; Okumura, K; Inoue, J; Watanabe, T. Tumor necrosis factor receptor-associated factor (TRAF)5 and TRAF2 are involved in CD30-mediated NFkB activation. *J Biol Chem,* 1997 272,2042-2045.

[17] Ellis, TM; Simms, PE; Slivnick, DJ; Jack, HM; Fisher, RI. CD30 is a signal-transducing molecule that defines a subsets of human activated CD45RO+ T cells. *Immunol,* 1993 151,2380-2389.

[18] Del Prete, G; De Carli, M; D'Elios, MM; Daniel, KC; Almerigogna, F; Alderson, M; Smith, CA; Thomas, E; Romagnani, S. CD30-mediated signals promotes the development of human helper type 2-like T cells. *J Exp Med,* 1995 182,1655-1661.

[19] Latza, U; Davis, S; Wilhelm, D; McKnight, B; Seyfarth, M; Stein, H. Soluble cytokine receptor CD30 in atopic disorders: a case-control study. *Clin Exp Allergy,* 1999 29,97-104.

[20] Okumura, M; Hidaka, Y; Matsuzuka, F. CD30 expression and interleukin-4 and intereron-γ production of intrathyroidal lymphocytes in Graves' disease. *Thyroid,* 1999 9,333-9.

[21] Iwagaki, H; Hizuta, A; Kohka, H; Kobashi, K; Nitta, Y; Isozaki, H; Takakura, N; Tanaka, N. Circulating levels of soluble CD30 and other markers in colorectal cancer patients. *J Med,* 1999 30,111-121.

[22] Nakamura, T; Lee, RK; Nam, SY; Al-Ramadi, BK; Koni, PA; Bottomly, K; Podack, ER; Flavell, RA. Reciprocal regulation of CD30 expression on CD4+ T cells by IL-4 and IFNγ. *J Immunol*, 1997 158,2090-2098.
[23] Pinto, A; Aldinucci, D; Gloghini, A; Zagonel, V; Degan, M; Improta, S; Juzbasic, S; Todesco, M; Perin, V; Gattei, V; Herrmann, F; Gruss, HJ; Carbone, A. Human eosinophils express functional CD30 ligand and stimulate proliferation of a Hodkin's disease cell line. *Blood*, 1996 88,3299-3305.
[24] Martinez, OM; Villaneuva, J; Abtahi, S; Beatty, PR; Esquivel, CO; Krams, SM. CD30 expression identifies a functional alloreactive human T-lymphocyte subset. *Transplantation*, 1998 65,1240-1247.
[25] Horie, R; Watanabe, T. CD30: expression and function in healt and disease. *Semin Immunol*, 1998 10,457-470.
[26] Matsumoto, K; Terakawa, M; Miura, K; Nakajima, T; Saito, H. Extremely rapid and intense induction of apoptosis in human eosinophils by anti-CD30 antibody treatment *in vitro*. *J Immunol*, 2004 172,2186-2193.
[27] Bloom, BR; Salgame, P; Diamond, B. Revisiting and revising suppressor T cells. *Immunol Today*, 1992 3,131-6.
[28] Cher, DJ; Mosmann, TR. Two types of murine helper T cell clones. II. Delayed-type hypersensitivity is mediated by TH1 clones. *J Immunol*, 1987 138,3688-94.
[29] Stevens, TL; Bossie, A; Sanders, WM; Fernandez-Botram, R; Coffman, LR; Mosmann, RT; Vitetta, ES. Regulation of antibody isotype secretion by subsets of antigen-specific helper T cells. *Nature*, 1988 334,255-8.
[30] Mosmann, TR; Schumacher, JH; Street, NF; Budd, R; O'Gara, A; Fong, TAT; Bond, MW; Moore, KWM; Sher, A; Fiorentino, DF. Diversity of cytokine synthesis and function of mouse $CD4^+$ T cells. *Immunol Rev*, 1991 123,209-29.
[31] Coffman, RL; Varkila, K; Scott, P; Chatelain, R. Role of cytokines in the differentiation of $CD4^+$ T-cell subsets *in vivo*. *Immunol Rev*, 1991 123,189-207.
[32] Peltz, G. A role for $CD4^+$ T cell subsets producing a selective pattern of lymphokines in the pathogenesis of human chronic inflammatory and allergic diseases. *Immunol Rev*, 1991 123,23-35.
[33] Murray, JS; Madri, J; Pasqualini, T; Bottomly, K. Functional CD4 T cell subset interplay in an intact immune system. *J Immunol*, 1993 150,4270-6.
[34] Thomson, AW; Dinarello, CA; Goldsmith, MA; Greene, WC; Bancherau, J; Rybak, ME; Hirano, T; Mosman, TR; De Maeyer, E; De Maeyer-Guignard, J; Tracey, KS; Pugh-Humphreys, RGP. In: Thomson A. (ed.) Academic press inc. *The cytokine handbook*. San Diego, CA; 1994.
[35] Kopf, M; Le Gros, G; Bachmann, M; Lamers, MC; Bluethmann, H; Köhler, G. Disruption of the murine IL-4 gene blocks TH2 cytokine responses. *Nature*, 1993 362,245-8.
[36] Tanaka, T; Hu-Li, J; Seder, RA; Fazekas de St.Groth, B; Paul, WE. Interleukin 4 suppresses interleukin 2 and interferon ### production by naive T cells stimulated by accessory cell-dependent receptor engagement. *Proc Natl Acad Sci USA*, 1993 90,5914-8.
[37] Bradley, LM; Yoshimoto, K; Swain, SL. The cytokines IL-4, IFN-gamma, and IL-12 regulate the development of subsets of memory effector helper T cells *in vitro*. *J Immunol*, 1995 155,1713-24.

[38] Banchereau, J. Converging and diverging properties of human interleukin-4 and interleukin-10. *Behring Institute Mitteilungen*, 1995 96,58-77.

[39] Fossa, SD; Aamdal, S; Naume, B; Gallati, H. Serum levels of cytokines and soluble cytokines receptors in patients with metastatic renal cell carcinoma or malignant melanoma receiving IL-2 interferon-alpha combination therapy. *Acta Oncol*, 1995 34,599-603.

[40] Lopez, M; Dilauro, L; Paoletti, G; Santini, S; Grandolfo, GM; Vitelli, G; Sfrasca, AM; Ameglio, F; Rasi, G; Garaci, E. Sequential biochemotherapy for metastatic colorectal cancer using fluorouracil, folinic acid, thymopentin and interleukin-2-clinical and immunological effects. *Annals Oncol*, 1995 6,1011-7.

[41] Wasik, MA; Vonderheid, EC; Bigler, RD; Marti, R; Lessin, SR; Polansky, M; Kadin, ME. Increased serum concentration of the soluble interleukin-2 receptor in cutaneous T-cell lymphoma-clinical and prognostic implications. *Arch Dermatol*, 1996 132,42-7.

[42] Kalinski, P; Vieira, PL; Schuitemaker, JK; De Jong, EC; Kapsenberg, ML. Prostaglandin E(2) is a selective inducer of interleukin-12 p40 (IL-12p40) production and an inhibitor of bioactive IL-12p70 heterodimer. *Blood*, 2001 97,3466-9.

[43] Costa, GL; Sandora, MR; Nakajima, A; Nguyen, EV; Taylor-Edwards, C; Slavin, AJ; Contag, CH; Fathman, CG; Benson, JM. Adoptive immunotherapy of experimental autoimmune encephalomyelite via T cell delivery of the IL-12 p40 subunit. *J Immunol*, 2001 167,2379-87.

[44] Acerwenka, A; Swain, SL. TGF-β1: immunosuppressant and viability factor for T lymphocytes. *Microbes and Infection*, 1999 15,1291-96.

[45] Lucey, DR; Clerici, M; Shearer, GM. Type 1 and type 2 cytokine dysregulation in human infectious, neoplastic, and inflammatory diseases. *Clin Microbiol Rev*, 1996 9,532-62.

[46] Pellegrini, P; Berghella, AM; Contasta, I; Adorno, D. CD30 antigen: not a physiological marker for TH2 cells but an important costimulator molecule in the regulation of the balance between TH1/TH2 response. *Transplant Immunology*, 2003 12,49-61.

[47] Hart, DNJ. Dendritic cells: Unique Leukocyte populations which control the primary immune response. *Blood*, 1997 90,3245-3287.

[48] Woodhead, BK. From sentinel to messenger: an extended phenotypic analysis of the monocyte to dendritic cells transition. *Immunology*, 1998 94,552-559.

[49] Huang, YM; Stoyanova, N; Jin, YP; Teleshova, N; Hussien, Y; Xiao, BG; Fredrikson, S; Link, H. Altered phenotype and function of blood dendritic cells in multiple sclerosis are modulated by IFN-β and IL-10. *Clin Exp Immunol*, 2001 124,306-14.

[50] Huang, YM; Kouwenhoven, M; Jin, YP; Press, R; Huang, WX; Link, H. Dendritic cells derived from patients with multiple sclerosis show high CD1a and low CD86 expression. *Mult Scler*, 2001 7,95-9.

[51] Duddy, ME; Dickson, G; Hawkins, SA; Armstrong, MA. Monocyte-derived dendritic cells: a potential target for therapy in multiple sclerosis (MS). *Clin Exp Immunol*, 2001 123,280-7.

[52] Berghella, AM; Totaro, R; Pellegrini, P; Contasta, I; Russo, T; Carolei, A; Adorno, D. Immunological study of IFNβ-1a treated and untreated Multiple Sclerosis patients: to

clarify IFNβ mechanisms and establish specific dendritic cell immunotherapy. *Neuroimmunomodulation*, 2005 (in press).
[53] Weinshenker, BG; Bass, B; Rice, GP; Noseworthy, J; Carriere, W; Baskerville, J; Ebers, GC. The natural history of multiple sclerosis: a geographically based study. I. Clinical course and disability. *Brain*, 1989 112,133-46.
[54] Weinshenker, BG; Bass, B; Rice, GP; Noseworthy, J; Carriere, W; Baskerville, J; Ebers, GC. The natural history of multiple sclerosis: a geographically based study. 2. Predictive value of the early clinical course. *Brain*, 1989 112,1419-28,
[55] Weinshenker, BG. Epidemiology of multiple sclerosis. *Neurol Clin*, 1996 14,291-308.
[56] Ferguson, B; Matyszak, MK; Esiri, MM; Perry, VH. Axonal damage in acute multiple sclerosis lesions. *Brain*, 1997 120,393-9.
[57] Chofflon, M; Ben-Amor, AF. Long-term benefits of early and high doses of interferon beta-1a treated ing multiple sclerosis. *Clin Neurol Neurosurg*, 2002 104,244-8.
[58] IFNB Multiple Sclerosis Study Group:Interferon beta-1b is effective in relapsing remitting multiple sclerosis. I. Clinical results of a multicenter, randomized, double-blind, placebo-controlled trial. *Neurology*, 1993 43,655-61.
[59] IFNB Multiple Sclerosis Study Group and the University of British Columbia MS/MRI Analysis Group: Interferon beta-1b in the treatment of multiple sclerosis: final outcome of the randomized controlled trial. *Neurology*, 1995 45,1277-85.
[60] Jacobs, LD; Cookfair, DL; Rudick, RA; Herndon, RM; Richert, JR; Salazar, AM; Fischer, JS; Goodkin, DE; Granger, CV; Simon, JH; Alam, JJ; Bartoszak, DM; Bourdette, DN; Braiman, J; Brownscheidle, CM; Coats, ME; Cohan, SL; Dougherty, DS; Kinkel, RP; Mass, MK; Munschauer, FE 3rd; Priore, RL; Pullicino, PM; Scherokman, BJ; Whitham, RH. Intramuscular interferon beta-1a for disease progression in relapsing multiple sclerosis. The Multiple Sclerosis Collaborative Research Group (MSCRG) *Ann Neurol*, 1996 39,285-94.
[61] Rudick, RA; Goodkin, DE; Jacobs LD; Cookfair, DL; Herndon, RM; Richert, JR; Salazar, AM; Fischer, JS; Granger, CV; Simon, JH; Alam, JJ; Simonian, NA; Campion, MK; Bartoszak, DM; Bourdette, DN; Braiman, J; Brownscheidle, CM; Coats, ME; Cohan, SL; Dougherty, DS; Kinkel, RP; Mass, MK; Munschauer, FE; Priore, RL; Whitham, RH. Impact of interferon beta-1a on neurologic disability in relapsing multiple sclerosis. The Multiple Sclerosis Collaborative Research Group (MSCRG). *Neurology*, 1997 49,358-63.
[62] PRISMS Study Group and the University of British Columbia MS/MRI Analysis Group.PRISMS-4:Long-term efficacy of interferon-beta-1a in relapsing MS. *Neurology*, 2001 56,1628-1636.
[63] Runkel, L; Meier, W; Pepinsky, RB; Karpusas, M; Whitty, A; Kimball, K; Brickelmaier, M; Muldowney, C; Jones, W; Goelz, SE. Structural and functional differences between glycosylated and non-glycosylated forms of human interferon-beta (IFN-beta). *Pharm Res*, 1998 15,641-9.
[64] Pellegrini, P; Totaro, R; Contasta, I; Berghella, AM; Carolei, A; Adorno, D. CD30 antigen and Multiple Sclerosis: CD30 an important costimulator molecule and marker for a regulatory subpopulation of dendritic cells involved in maintaining the physiological balance between TH1/TH2 immune response and tollerance; the role of

IFNβ-1a in re-establishing this regulation in Multiple Sclerosis. *Neuroimmunol*, (in press) 2005
[65] Hargreaves, PG; Al-Shamkhani, A. Soluble CD30 bloks transmembrane signaling by CD30. *Eur J Immunol*, 2002 32.163-173.
[66] Susal, C; Pelzl, S; Simon, T; Opelz, G. Advances in pre- and posttransplant immunologic testing in kidney trasplantation. *Transplant Proc*, 2004 36,29-34.
[67] Zanotti, R; Trolese, A; Ambrosetti, A; Nadali, G; Visco, C; Ricetti, MM; Benedetti, F; Pizzolo, G. Serum levels of soluble CD30 improve International prognostic score in predicting the outcome of advanced Hodgkin's lymphoma. *Annals Oncol*, 2002 13,1908-1914.
[68] Rose, NR. Autoimmunity at a turning point: from investigation to intervention. *Autoimmunity Reviews*, 2002 1,3-4.
[69] Kurt, C; Carbone, FR; Krummel, MF; Kock, MK; Miller, JF; Heath, WR. Signalling trough CD30 protects against autoimmune diabetes mediated by CD8 T cells. *Nature*, 1999 398,341a5.
[70] French, MA; Lewin, SR; Dykstra, C; Krueger, R; Price, P; Leedman, Pj. Graves' disease during immune reconstitution after higly active antiretroviral therapy for HIV infection: evidence of thymic dysfunction. *AIDS Res Hum Retrovirus*, 2004 20,157-162.
[71] Sakaguchi, S; Sakaguchi, N; Asano, M; Itoh, M; Toda, M. Immunologic self-tolerance maintained by activated T cells expressing IL-2 receptor alpha-chains (CD25). Break down of a single mechanism of self-tolerance causes various autoimmune diseases. *J Immunol*, 1995 155,1151-1164
[72] Compston, A; Coles, A. Multiple Sclerosis. *The Lancet*, 2002 359,1221-1231.
[73] Lassmann, H; Bruck, W; Lucchinetti, C. Heterogeneity of multiple sclerosis pathogenesis: implications for diagnosis and therapy. *Trends Mol Med*, 2001 7,115-21.
[74] Merrill, JE. Proinflammatory and antiinflammatory cytokines in multiple sclerosis and central nervous system acquired immunodeficiency syndrome. *J Immunother*, 1992 12,167-70.
[75] Sorensen, TL; Tani, M; Jensen, J; Pierce, V; Lucchinetti, C; Folcik, VA; Qin, S; Rottman, J; Sellebjerg, F; Strieter, RM; Frederiksen, JL; Ransohoff, RM. Expression of specific chemokines and chemokine receptors in the central nervous system of multiple sclerosis patients. *J Clin Invest*, 1999 103,807-15.
[76] Mason, D. A very high level of crossreactivity is an essential feature of the T-cell receptor. *Immunol Today*, 1998 19,395-404.
[77] Sprent, J; Kishimoto, H. The thymus and negative selection. *Inmmunol Rev*, 2002 185,126-135.
[78] Seddon, B; Mason, D. The third function of the thymus. *Immunol Today*, 2000 21,95-99.
[79] Papiernik, M; De Moraes, ML; Pontoux, C; Vasseur, F; Penit, C. Regulatory CD4 T cells: expression of IL-2R alpha chain, resistance to clonal deletion and IL-2 dependency. *Int. Immunol*, 1998 10,371-378.
[80] Schevach, EM. Certified professionals: CD4(+)CD25(+) suppressor T cells. *J Exp Med*, 2001 193,F41-6.

[81] Levings, MK; Sangregorio, R; Roncarolo, MG. Human cd25(+)cd4(+) t regulatory cells suppress naive and memory T cell proliferation and can be expanded *in vitro* without loss of function. *J Exp Med*, 2001 193,1295-302.
[82] Thornton, AM; Shevach, EM. CD4+CD25+ immunoregulatory T cells suppress polyclonal T cell activation *in vitro* by inhibiting interleukin 2 production. *J Exp Med*, 1998 188,287-96.
[83] Jonuleit, H; Schmitt, E; Stassen, M; Tuettenberg, A; Knop, J; Enk, AH. Identification and functional characterization of human CD4(+)CD25(+) T cells with regulatory properties isolated from peripheral blood. *J Exp Med*, 2001 193,1285-94.
[84] Dieckmann, D; Plottner, H; Berchtold, S; Berger, T; Schuler, G. Ex vivo isolation and characterization of CD4(+)CD25(+) T cells with regulatory properties from human blood. *J Exp Med*, 2001 193,1303-10.
[85] Ng, WF; Duggan, PJ; Ponchel, F; Matarese, G; Lombardi, G; Edwards, AD; Isaacs, JD; Lechler, RI. Human CD4(+)CD25(+) cells: a naturally occurring population of regulatory T cells. *Blood*, 2001 98,2736-44
[86] Seddon, B; Mason, D. Peripheral autoantigen induces regulatory T cells that prevent autoimmunity. *J Exp Med*, 1999 189,877-82.
[87] Taams, LS; Smith, J; Rustin, MH; Salmon, M; Poulter, LW; Akbar, AN. Human anergic/suppressive CD4(+)CD25(+) T cells: a highly differentiated and apoptosis-prone population. *Eur J Immunol*, 2001 31,1122-31.
[88] Read, S; Malmstrom, V; Powrie, F. Cytotoxic T lymphocyte-associated antigen 4 plays an essential role in the function of CD25(+)CD4(+) regulatory cells that control intestinal inflammation. *J Exp Med*, 2000 192,295-302.
[89] Takahashi, T; Tagami, T; Yamazaki, S; Uede, T; Shimizu, J; Sakaguchi, N; Mak, TW; Sakaguchi, S. Immunologic self-tolerance maintained by CD25(+)CD4(+) regulatory T cells constitutively expressing cytotoxic T lymphocyte-associated antigen 4. *J Exp Med*, 2000 192,303-10.
[90] McHugh, RS; Whitters, MJ; Piccirillo, CA; Young, DA; Shevach, EM; Collins, M; Byrne, MC. CD4(+)CD25(+) immunoregulatory T cells: gene expression analysis reveals a functional role for the glucocorticoid-induced TNF receptor. *Immunity*, 2002 16,311-23.
[91] Shimizu, J; Yamazaki, S; Takahashi, T; Ishida, Y; Sakaguchi, S. Stimulation of CD25(+)CD4(+) regulatory T cells through GITR breaks immunological self-tolerance. *Nat Immunol*, 2002 3,135-42.
[92] Jonuleit, H; Adema, G; Schmitt, E. Immune regulation by regulatory T cells: implications for transplantation. *Transpl Immunol*, 2003 11,267-76.
[93] Jonuleit, H; Schmitt, E; Kakirman, H; Stassen, M; Knop, J; Enk, AH. Infectious tolerance: human CD25(+) regulatory T cells convey suppressor activity to conventional CD4(+) T helper cells. *J Exp Med*, 2002 196,255-60.
[94] Dieckmann, D; Bruett, CH; Ploettner, H; Lutz, MB; Schuler, G. Human CD4(+)CD25(+) regulatory, contact-dependent T cells induce interleukin 10-producing, contact-independent type 1-like regulatory T cells. *J Exp Med*, 2002 196,247-53.
[95] Bloemena, E; Roos, MT; Van Heijst, JL; Vossen, JM; Schellekens, PT. Whole-blood lymphocyte cultures. *J Immunol Methods*, 1989 122,161-7.

[96] Syrjala, H; Herva, E; Ilonen, J; Saukkonen, K; Salminen, A. A whole-blood lymphocyte stimulation test for the diagnosis of human tularemia. *J Infect Dis*, 1984 150,912-303.

[97] Muller, K; Herner, EB; Stagg, A; Bendtzen, K; Woo, P. Inflammatory cytokines and cytokine antagonists in whole blood cultures of patients with systemic juvenile chronic arthritis. *Br J Rheumatol*, 1998 37,562-9.

[98] Berghella, AM; Pellegrini, P; Piancatelli, D; Maccarone, D; Del Beato, T; Giubilei, D; Pomidori, A; Adorno, D; Casciani, CU. Progression mechanisms in colon cancer: soluble interleukin-2 (IL-2) receptor, IL-2 plus anti-CD3 proliferative response and tumour stage correlations. *Cancer Immunol Immunother*, 1994 38,160-166.

[99] Bridoux, F; Badou, A; Saoudi, A; Bernard, I; Druet, E; Pasquier, R; Druet, P; Pelletier, L: Transforming growth factor beta (TGF-beta)-dependent inhibition of T helper cell 2 (Th2)-induced autoimmunity by self-major histocompatibility complex (MHC) class II-specific, regulatory CD4(+) T cell lines. *J Exp Med*, 1997 185,1769-75.

[100] Shinomiya, M; Fazle Akbar, SM; Shinomiya, H; Onji, M. Transfer of dendritic cells (DC) ex vivo stimulated with interferon-gamma (IFN-gamma) down-modulates autoimmune diabetes in non-obese diabetic (NOD) mice. *Clin Exp Immunol*, 1999 117,38-43.

[101] Jin, YX; Xu, LY; Guo, H; Ishikawa, M; Link, H; Xiao, BG. TGF-beta1 inhibits protracted-relapsing experimental autoimmune encephalomyelitis by activating dendritic cells. *J Autoimmun*, 2000 14,213-20.

[102] Fukao, T; Frucht, DM; Yap, G; Gadina, M; O'Shea, JJ; Koyasu, S. Inducible expression of Stat4 in dendritic cells and macrophages and its critical role in innate and adaptive Immune responses. *J Immunol*, 2001 166,4446-55.

[103] Chomarat, P; Banchereau, J; Davoust, J; Palucka, AK. IL6 switches the differentiation of monocytes from dendritic cells to macrophages. *Nat Immunol*, 2000 1,510-4.

[104] Menetrier-Caux, C; Thomachot, MC; Alberti, L; Montmain, G; Blay, JY. IL-4 prevents the blockade of dendritic cell differentiation induced by tumor cells. *Cancer Res*, 2001 61,3096-104.

[105] Berghella, AM; Pellegrini, P; Del Beato, T; Marini, M; Tomei, E; Adorno, D; Casciani, CU. The significance of an increase in soluble interleukin-2 receptor level in colorectal cancer and its biological regulating role in the physiological switching of the immune response cytokine network from TH1 to TH2 and back. *Cancer Immunol Immunother*, 1998 45,241-249

[106] Del Beato, T; Berghella, AM; Pellegrini, P; Adorno, D; Casciani, CU. The role of the soluble CD30 serum level in colorectal cancer: a possible marker for a patient subset which could benefit from IL-2 biotherapy. *Cancer Biother & Radiopharmaceuticals*, 1997 12,297-304.

In: Multiple Sclerosis Research Progress
Editors: H. Schwarz, L. Walter
ISBN: 978-1-60456-570-6
© 2008 Nova Science Publishers, Inc.

Chapter 7

INVISIBLE BODIES: OLDER WOMEN AND MULTIPLE SCLEROSIS

Louise Dawson
University of Central Lancashire, Pieston, Lancashire, UK

INTRODUCTION

This chapter explores the relationship between older women and the lived experience of Multiple Sclerosis (MS). The paper investigates the narratives of the women living with MS and presents them as critical insights into current health-care provision in the UK. Influenced by post-structuralist discourse analysis and the work of Michael Foucault, this chapter reflects the importance of representing the power relations constituted in discourse, particularly through the body via medical discursive regimes (Turner 1992). The experience of women's disciplined bodies over time is discussed within a context of multiple subjectivities and the 'real life' health inequalities. For example, the author juxtaposes the illness stories of the women living with MS with their historical and contemporary recollections of health-care. The author argues that the experience of healthcare for these older women's bodies has been influenced by the gender regimes imposed by medical authority. This chapter raises questions within and around women and neurology specifically using Multiple Sclerosis to understand the experience of women's ageing bodies.

MS is a disease of the central nervous system and is an umbrella term for a wide range of symptoms (Sibley, 1988). The most common symptoms are fatigue, visual problems, pain, stiffness and spasms, depression, cognitive problems, speech problems, continence issues and sexual problems (Perry, 1994). It is predominantly experienced by women with a current ratio of 3:2 (MS Society UK, 2005). Currently there is no known cure for MS and no generally agreed definition of the origins of disease (Halper and Holland, 1997; Burgess, 2002).

This research is based on the author's own studies into the life trajectories of women living with a diagnosis of Multiple Sclerosis. The research has been carried out over a six year period and has evolved within a process of research reflections, specifically as the author draws on her own experiences of living with MS. Overall seventeen interviews were carried out with women who had a diagnosis of MS and the ages of the women ranged from twenty-one to seventy-three. Supplementary data was collected through thirty written life histories provided by women with MS (see Berrey, 2003, for further information on life history approaches). This chapter focuses on older women with MS, with the term older being defined as women over fifty. However, in some parts the voice of Jesse aged twenty one, and some other younger women, are used to juxtapose the experiences of age and explore some conceptual issues such as body surveillance and control through time and space. The data collection was analysed using a framework of narrative analysis, drawing on temporality, to explore their experiences of illness over time (Koch, 1998; Ochs and Capps, 1996). Within this framework the author explores many of the medical inscriptions placed on women's bodies and how these have impacted on women's experiences of illness. This chapter is based on the initial findings from doctoral research and is part of work in progress.

Arthur Frank (1995) discusses in his book 'The Wounded Storytelller' (based on research about people with cancer) how people who experience illness, both short term and long term, need to make sense of what is happening to them. This chapter presents women with MS as wounded storytellers and explores their narratives to understand the lived experience of disease. The wounded body can be an empowering experience as it can provide a voice to express beyond the physical limitations (Barrett 1995; Stacey 1997). Frank (1995) and Stacey (1997) recognise that stories of illness empower the teller in several ways. Firstly, the person telling the story becomes a creator of knowledge through discussing their experiences (Koch, 1998). By doing so, they can become recognised within their experience and provide insight and common sense understanding to people in similar situations (Capps, 1996; Koch, 1998). When somebody has been disempowered through an experience of illness, certain types of knowledge within and around the illness can provide empowerment (Bruner, 1987; Frank, 1995). This chapter will explore the women's narratives of their illness stories and offer another way to understand the complexities hidden within them. Firstly a discussion of the medical inscriptions placed on women's bodies will precede a more detailed discussion of older women living with MS. This will explore the women's temporal experiences and suggest some inequalities of healthcare for them. This will then be summarised with some suggestions for the future of older women living with MS.

History of Women's Bodies

Patients play a certain role in reproducing the hierarchies of medical authority (Frank 1995). Individuals, specifically women, engage with healthcare through a certain set of rules and regulations such as establishing themselves as patients via a health centre or hospital (Foster, 1995). The theatre of hospital requires role playing with multiple agencies dependant on people displaying certain beliefs, behaviours and practices. The structural functioning of hospitals and medical houses are based on routine, established practise, and care (Stacey, 1997). Certainly, any ill-health in the Western world involves a medical construct imposed in order to surveil the well and unwell body routinely (Sontag, 1991).

Feminists have contributed to this debate recognising the pathologisation of women's bodies in the current healthcare system and the dominance of this in the cultural understandings of disease for women (Ussher, 1992; Lupton, 1994). For example, Bush (2000) emphasises the cultural practise of cervical smears to modify and then inform women about certain aspects of their sexuality, so inscribing a particular responsibility onto them. This can be seen in many of the health practices ascribed onto women's health through discursive regimes and gendered medical knowledges (Foster, 1995; Nettleton, 1995). In recent years much health research for women has focused on challenging the issues around and within reproductive health (Martin, 1989; Roberts, 2000). Currently feminists have been identifying other areas of health concern for women, such as disability and learning difficulties, establishing the multiple differences within women's health experiences (Vanselow, 2000).

Historically the male body has been viewed as the norm, and women by definition are regarded as inherently deviant (Ussher, 1991; Vanselow, 2000). Female behaviour that may be perplexing to the male view has been attributed to physiology rather than women's position in society (Martin, 1989). Comparisons have been drawn between the nineteenth century diagnosis of hysteria and the contemporary reproductive syndromes of Premenstrual Syndrome (PMS), post-natal depression and menopause as expressions of social powerlessness rather than illness (Ussher, 1992). Elaine Showalter (1987), discusses the importance of morality in the history of madness and emphasises the contextualisation of this in reference to the Victorian management of insanity underpinned by the ethos of self-control (see Showalter, 1987). Martin (1989) contextualises the reproductive systems of women as being heavily inscribed with gendered stereotypes. Martin (1989) analyses the discursive practices of women's bodies and outlines how these become culturally understood as an interpretive reflection and inscription of gender dynamics. This can be located as a historical emergence of gender identity with dominant discourses such as madness and hysteria being identified to explain women's subordination. McNay (1994) applies these issues to women's bodies and the surveillance of women through discourse that controls, subordinates and impinges on their lived experience.

OLDER WOMEN LIVING WITH MS

There is a distinct gap in MS related literature that denies acknowledgment of older women's self-perspectives (Burgess 2002). The studies that focus around this topic are predominantly quality of life (QOL) studies that are derived from biomedical model understandings of the body, with most studies segregating the lived experience of disease (Perry, 1994). Any studies that claim to be based on experience are still within the parameters of the biomedical model and they suggest a 'truth' about the body (Barrett, 1995). Most of the qualitative literature that researches MS experiences is done using a multi-disciplinary approach and significantly takes on medical assumptions around care experiences (Halper and Holland, 1997). The few studies relating to older women with MS focus on bladder and bowel problems, diverting the conversation to that of practical constraints (Perry, 1994). Very few current qualitative studies look at the experience of MS for older women outside of the biomedical model. For example Barrett (1995) explores the diagnosis of MS for women using anthropological understandings of the body and critiques the influences of the biomedical understandings of the body but looks at the experiences of women as a group rather than using age as a differing experience. Also, few suggest the body as being socially engaged but merely as an entity that is viewed in a medicalised way (Barrett, 1995). Other studies surrounding MS focus on particular issues, such as coping with symptoms, addressing practical concerns, but most fail to understand or challenge the bodily experience due to their over reliance a biomedical view of the world (See Burgess 2002 for an overview of current qualitative studies for women with MS).

Older women living with Multiple Sclerosis have largely remained invisible within the discourses of health, particularly in the current literature and more specifically in the long term plans for neurological healthcare (Go to http://www.mssociety.org.uk for an overview of current funded projects) Current research looking at MS tends to focus on younger people and provide hope for new treatment plans. The health literature for older people tends to focus towards care and need, initiating an acceptance of disease progression. Older women become visible at certain points in the literature such as alleviating incontinence problems, but are discursively excluded from research developments in science which narrate cause and cure.

Women Living with MS: Age as a Difference

The ages of the women in the study ranged from twenty to seventy-one, and the research identified a significant difference and inequality in their healthcare experiences dependant on age. Taking into account the structural and economic disadvantage experienced by women over time, the younger women interviewed tended to engage with medical authority from a higher level of awareness about their bodies. Several of the younger women interviewed discussed their relationship with medical professionals in a critical way and had challenged the knowledges they had been presented with.

> I strongly oppose the idea that doctors throw anti-depressants at women with MS. Whatever my beliefs into what and how the disease originates I get very cross that these zombie drugs are offered about. I do tell the doctor though so he knows my view and I must say he does respect it. It's very important to take a stand on these issues, it really is (Jesse aged 21).

This is one example from the younger group of women who were interviewed. Jesse's narrative above reflected the opinions of the other younger women who were also interviewed. The general understanding of the younger group of women was that of critical awareness on medical practices. Louise (aged 21) agreed with Jesse's viewpoint suggesting that women with MS need to take particular care when deciding what drugs to take due to the 'unmonitored' approach. The most common forms of treatment for MS until recently have been anti-depressant drugs and sedative grouped drugs, an issue which has come under scrutiny over the past five years (Burgess, 2002; MS Society, 2005). The challenging discourses of the younger women were enhanced by their obvious critique of medical knowledge and informed approach to their healthcare. For example Louise said:

> I know that doctors can be extremely gendered in their approach to healthcare for women but as a young woman training to be a nurse I know that I am more than capable of challenging the traditional models that dominate some medical perceptions. I also know that MS is a puzzle to most medical doctors and that is why I choose to explore alternative routes to take care of myself.

For the younger women interviewed a critical reflexive approach to their bodies and medicine was discernable in the stories they told of their health experiences. They did not feel oppressed or inscribed in the medical regimes offered to them because they felt in control of their health. Several of the younger women commented that they used the healthcare system to 'dip in and out off' as they felt they had a good understanding of their bodies and MS. This was an immediate awareness for them whereas the older women experienced medical regimes and practices over periods of time before they developed their own personal awareness. The older women discursively showed an awareness of their bodies that had been a gradual process over a number of years and had developed through their engagement with medical regimes over a period of time also. All of the older women discussed their experiences with medical professionals as a changing relationship which they identified as being located in particular times and spaces. As highlighted by Elsie (aged 66):

> Years ago I respected doctors. Now I distrust them. If I know them, than I'm ok but put me in a room with a strange neurologist for example and I would just shut up. Either that or walk out because they are mostly arrogant and when you get old, like me, they are just not interested. They are waiting for you to die.

SUBJECTIVE IDENTITIES FOR OLDER WOMEN

The author talked to more than ten women who were aged over fifty. The older women discussed their issues with disability over time and talked about a period of adjustment. This was very much dictated by their experiences with health professionals. However, there were differences in the levels of authority, for example, the women talked about relationships with nurses more easily than those with doctors. They were also more likely to challenge nurses and social workers but had a level of acceptance about the information given to them by doctors and neurologists. However, sometimes this manifested as a feeling of intimidation linked to perceived status and class of the doctors and neurologists. They felt more comfortable to ask questions to nurses, and felt that social workers should be questioned. This was identified by three main themes discussed by the women. These focused around symptoms, diagnosis and their emotional responses to their own particular health experiences.

Symptoms

All of the older women interviewed had experienced symptoms of MS for a significant number of years before a diagnosis had been made. It is important to remember that the symptoms experienced by the women ranged from numbness and loss of co-ordination in either their arms or legs; bladder and bowel control; a range of motor symptoms such as slurred speech; cognitive deficiencies; and partial or total loss of sight.

All of the women had been told they had anxiety problems and their symptoms had been related to issues of hormones - particularly as all the older women had children.

> When I had my first child I started having blurred eyesight and suffered with funny legs. You know what I mean, weak and wobbly, sometimes I thought I was going to fall over. The

> doctor said that when you have children it changes your body and that's how he explained it (Sally aged 63).

Most of the women could trace their first symptoms back to their early twenties and each was over fifty before MS was confirmed. They had spent many years battling with the symptoms of MS, usually explained as a hormonal or anxiety problem.

> Doctors said it was me hormones and that, so you just take what they give you at first and you don't question. Why would I? In my day women didn't question (Iris aged 71).

This lack of questioning was a common theme among all the women and they had accepted their GP's diagnosis that hormonal changes had caused the symptoms they had been experiencing. The women also described experiencing symptoms after each child they gave birth too which again was defined as hormonal problems without further investigation.

> With each child I was always ill afterwards. Not when I was pregnant, usually I was alright for nine months, but afterwards I always had the flu or something - my daughter who is a nurse now said she had read in a book that this happens to women with MS. They always blame women's hormones don't they? (Doris aged 67).

There is a growing body of research around MS and pregnancy that supports the view that hormone imbalance can effect the progression of MS (see Perry 1994). However, this information is presented as a supportive measure to women deciding to have children, and not as an oppressive issue that could subordinate their decision making over having a family (Perry, 1994). In relation to Doris's (see above) comment, research has shown that when women with MS are pregnant their health improves initially, but may decline after the birth. This is a finding in recent MS research (MS Society UK, 2005), and has developed due to more funding being concentrated on MS research for younger women. Most of the older women had been encouraged by their doctors not to have any more children once their symptoms developed, although the women were only told they had hormonal problems, depression and anxiety problems. Their doctors may have suspected MS was the cause of their symptoms, but whatever the cause, the women were not being given good information to make informed choices about their bodies.

Another common theme was the diagnosis of depression and anxiety to explain the women's symptoms. Some of the younger women had also experienced this but had actually challenged their doctors and insisted on further investigation. The older women had accepted this inscription of depression as they did not feel comfortable to challenge the doctor.

> I was put on tranquillisers years ago…too many to remember. The doctor just said I had anxiety and depression and he said the tranquilisers would relax me. I must admit, they stopped making me worry about the symptoms but it's not right is it to be spaced out for all them years? I do think I missed out on a lot with the kids because of this (Doreen aged 67).

All the older women had had a period where they had been placed on tranquillisers or anti-depressants for the symptoms they were experiencing. Some had been on strong medication for a period of twenty years, with most of them coming off it when they received an official diagnosis of MS.

Diagnosis

The women's stories of a diagnosis of MS all had a similar theme. All of the women had experienced symptoms of MS for a period of up to twenty years and held the belief that depression and anxiety had caused them. Symptoms of MS had been defined as hormonal problems, anxiety problems or depression by their GP's. Initially the women found a diagnosis of MS confusing and could not comprehend what had happened to them. Several of the women suggested they had accepted they were depressed and felt huge tensions about their bodies with a diagnosis of MS.

> For years I thought I was nervous-maybe I am I'm not sure, but to then find out it was something else, is something else, is frightening. Sometimes I get cross because I think "who are you (in reference to the GP) to decide what I've got ?"(Elsie, aged 66)

This tension was reflected by a number of stories told by the women. The women said they went through a period of shock that left them feeling disorientated.

> I mean what do you do with it? At first I thought they were saying I had something extra as well as anxiety, then they said it was probably all MS, then some cheeky young doctor said people with MS do get depressed-I said, well they could only get depressed if they knew about it! (Iris aged 71)

The women expressed their concern at experiencing symptoms for a number of years before a diagnosis of MS was given. Four of the women had since found out that a diagnosis of MS had been written on their medical records up to twenty years before they were told they had MS. These women had also found out that their husbands or partners had been told of their diagnosis but informed by the doctor not to tell them as this could accelerate their condition.

> When I got my diagnosis (she was 50 when told by a neurologist) it was casually given by this neurologist I had been sent to. I was really confused about it and a few years ago, you know, when it became legal to look at your doctor records, I got mine and they said 'suspected MS'-this had been written when I was in my twenties. I was really angry cause I since found out my ex-husband knew and the GP had told him not to mention it to me as they couldn't do anything about it (Colette aged 58).

The women explained that having MS did not cause the major concern, but they felt betrayed by their GPs and also let down by their partners and husbands who had been aware of their prognosis. On reflection they had felt like second class citizens and explained this in the context of their life experiences. For example, Elsie explained:

> I think what hurt the most was Eric knew and he never told me. Our whole marriage he used to ignore me and tell me I was mad - I now understand why. The bloody doctor had told him as much. I feel like my life has been a fraud for all them years...yeah, that hurts the most (Elsie aged 66).

Emotional Responses

The women expressed their emotional understandings of having a diagnosis of MS after experiencing symptoms for a period of years. They initially discussed the impact of believing they were depressed to discovering they actually had a neurological disorder. The women expressed feelings of anger, turmoil and betrayal at the medical system. They recounted numerous stories when they had felt ridiculed by health professionals when attempting to gain some clarity over their condition and their bodies.

> I remember being a young woman, about 27, and I had lost the feeling in my right arm and was limping in my right leg. I was so frightened as I thought I must have had a stroke or something. When I told the doctor he looked at me puzzled and asked how my periods were. I said they were fine - I ended up leaving his room with a bottle of pills to make me relax (Elsie, aged 66).

The women had approached their GP's with bladder problems and were told that problems with 'their waterworks' should be expected after having children. Over time the women eventually managed to get a referral to a neurologist. The women acknowledged this to be indicative of changing times for women and of becoming more valued and 'treated like a person'. Emotionally the experience had left the women drained. They felt that they had missed out on trying to get well by not knowing what had been wrong with them. The women also felt deceived at many levels and did feel like they had been exposed. Doreen said:

> It's a feeling of loss but one of exposure. They know what's wrong with you but choose to not tell until they want to. It's like a circus, a freak show, but we are meant to be good people in this country - aren't we?

All of the women had an understanding of what had caused 'their MS'. At the onset of disease all the women articulated some traumatic event to coincide with their first symptoms. Even at the early stage of disease the women recognised that a major personal circumstance had triggered their first attack. This was always an emotional encounter related to their immediate life course. Although this could be a build up of tension located in the women's life history, in the women's lives there was one major impact that they related to the onset of disease. Alice *(aged 67)* recalled:

> Getting diagnosed with MS actually gave me an 'opt out' from where I was at. At the time I was working so hard running one of the (families) guest houses - and I hated it. It was a twenty four hour job and it was very, very difficult. Being ill allowed me to think, be alone and assess where I was up to. That was ten years ago now and I haven't looked back.

Alice accepted her MS onset to be a reflection of her lifestyle at the time. She had previously been told she had anxiety for a number of years but related this to her unhappy life situation. The diagnosis of MS meant that she could evaluate her life and remove herself from some of the situations she had found herself in. Alice also felt that she did too many things to please other people and she wasn't being honest to herself.

Alice concluded:

> I consciously remember feeling a sense of achievement and acknowledgment when I lost the feeling in my right arm. I knew that my pain, the dull one in my stomach, was coming into show. I always knew that my MS was related to my life and all its drama.

These women had never been asked by any health professionals what they believed to be the cause of their MS. They had never been asked any questions about their healthcare and what choices they may or may not want to make. In the case of this research, it was the first time these older women with MS had been asked for their own opinion about their experience of MS.

Women Living with MS: Health Provisions

Despite the fact that many older women with MS find themselves receiving treatment of some kind for their symptoms, overall their healthcare is poor (Busfield, 2000). They have been, and continue to be, routinely discriminated against within primary care (Bartley, Blane and Davey Smith, 1998). Recent research into the general health provision of people with MS firmly identifies such inequality, with older women receiving minimum or total lack of support in terms of neurological provision (Burgess 2002). Through the construct of age the women have become discredited and ignored in terms of evaluating their own needs (Myers and Macdonald, 1996). This effects how they will engage in medical practise as for the most part they will be excluded from drug trials and new treatment plans. Women's experiences of MS and health-care are dependant on their particular geographical locations in the UK. The regional politics and disparities of health service distribution disadvantage some women and the economically marginalised. This post-code lottery, underpinned by issues of age, race, ethnicity and class amongst other disadvantages creates an unequal and discriminatory approach to receiving healthcare.

Dealing with the Professionals

The older women interviewed felt that healthcare for people with MS was generally poor in quality. They particularly felt that as they aged they became more excluded. The women also distrusted medical professionals through their experiences of mis-diagnosis. They had contradictory feelings towards doctors and neurologists and had more challenging and engaging relationships with nurses and social workers. All the women had a good relationship with their own current GPs but sometimes had problems with other hierarchical figures - particularly ones that they did not know very well.

> When I was in hospital for a chest infection they put me on the chest ward. I kept asking the doctor if I could see a neurologist because I knew that underneath everything it was my MS. Of course, low immune system is the central thing to MS but he wouldn't listen. In the end he told me to shut as he was in charge. I blame him for my limp now because it was that

night I had a bad attack and he just left me (Doreen aged 68 recalling an experience in hospital).

The majority of the older women had experienced tensions especially when they had been admitted to hospital. This was due to the lack of general knowledge about MS between health professionals and the women felt that there was no consistency between specialists. A few of the women thought this may be because of the lack of MS specialist centres. They also raised concern about the rules and regulations of access to health resources and felt there was a lack of communication between health workers.

> The social worker visited me at home to assess me for a wheelchair. My house is so small as you can see but she insisted I am only allowed an indoor one before I qualify for an outdoor one-so here I am still unable to go outside with an indoor wheelchair that's too big to use inside-what is the point of this? (Lorraine aged 55).

Some of the women felt that service provision lacked a humanitarian approach and did not take into account the women as people. This made them feel devalued as women.

> I find it difficult when Bob has to put me on the toilet. I asked the social worker for a home help assessment but she said no because Bob is my husband and that's that she said-is this right? (Jenny aged 57).

The women all held a good comprehensive knowledge of the healthcare system, particularly around service provision. Most of the older women said they would welcome the chance to change things in the health service - they just did not know how to do it. The women all said they had attempted to communicate their experiences to social workers but felt they had not been taken seriously. They wondered if this was because of their age or because they were disabled.

Conclusion: Women and MS

Gender research looking at women's experiences of MS is a much under- funded research area. Broadly speaking, more qualitative research is needed that looks at women's experiences of neurological problems from the perspective of the women's lives. A lot can be gained from starting research with subjective experiences of life, and as highlighted in this chapter, much can be learned from these experiences.

This chapter uses Multiple Sclerosis as an illustrative way of exploring health provision within a hegemonic healthcare system that heavily relies on the interpretations of illness as defined by medical discourses. As highlighted in this chapter, there is no known cause or cure for MS, yet the inscribed understanding of these older women's experiences reflects the gendered notions of hysteria from the Victorian era. The limitations of that knowledge undermines the agency of these women, and as can be seen from the illustrative studies used above, succeeded for a period of these women's lives. By assessing the women's temporal experiences the author suggests that a more detailed contribution to MS research exists in understanding MS through subjective experiences. This could provide a more caring and understanding approach for older women living with illness and protect other women from being tailored into a specific role that satisfies the dominance of the medical narrative in this area.

For the older women interviewed they felt they did not fit into the current healthcare system. Their position is not that of many other women wishing to challenge the patriarchal, Westernized construction of gender roles. Their battle with life and everyday living is much more concise and often desperate. The women's own stories of their health problems significantly suggest that the current medical, social and healthcare model of the National Health Service (NHS) does not reflect the real life experiences of these women - particularly older women – and consequently detracts from their support and treatment. There is a huge gulf between the medical discourses that address the challenges of MS and the lived recollection of their own experiences.

REFERENCES

Barrett, J. (1995), Multiple sclerosis; The Experience of a Disease. *Women's Studies International Forum* 18(2): 159-171.

Bartley, M; Blane, D. and Davey Smith, G. (1998), *The Sociology of Health Inequalities,* Blackwell Publsihers: Oxford.

Berrey, E. (2003), Life History: the integrity of her voice, In Clare, J. and Haidton, *Writing Research: Transforming Data into Research, Churchill Livingstone: Elsever Science.*

Bruner, J. (1987), Life a narrative. *Social Research 54: 11-32.*

Burgess, M (2002), *Multiple Sclerosis: Theory and Practice for nurses,* London, Whurr Publishers Ltd.

Busfield, J. (2000), *Health and Health Care in Modern Britain*, Oxford University Press: Oxford.

Bush, J (2000), "It's just part of being a woman": cervical screening, the body and femininity, *Social Science and Medicine,* 50(3): 429-444, February issue.

Foster, P (1995), *Women and the Health Care Industry. An Unhealthy Relationship?* Open University Press, Buckingham.

Frank, A. (1995), *The Wounded Storyteller: Body, Illness and Ethics*, The University of Chicago Press: Chicago and London.

Halper, J. and Holland, N. (1997), *Comprehensive Nursing Care in Multiple Sclerosis*, Demos Vermande: New York.

Koch, T. (1998), Story telling: is it really research? *Journal of Advanced Nursing, 28(6), 1182-1190.*

Lupton, D. (1994), *Medicine As Culture: Illness, Disease, and The Body in Western Societies.* London: Sage.

Martin, E. (1989), *The Woman in the Body: A Cultural Analysis of Reproduction,* Milton McNay Keynes: Open University Press.

Multiple Sclerosis Society http://www.mssociety.org.uk

McNay , L (1994), *Foucault: a critical introduction*, Cambridge, Polity Press.

Nettleton, S. (1995), *The Sociology of Health and Illness*, Polity Press: Cambridge.

Ochs, E. and Capps, L. (1996), Narrating The Self, *Annual Review of Anthropology*, 25:19-43.

Perry, S. (1994), *Living with Multiple Sclerosis: personal accounts of coping and adaption,* Ashgate Publishers: Aldershot.

Roberts, C. (2000), Sex Hormones As Biocultural Actors: Rethinking Biology, Sexual Difference And Health, In Ussher, J. (Eds) *Women's Health: Contemporary International Perspectives,* (pp. 283-290), BPS Books: Leicester.

Showalter, E. (1987), *The Female Malady: Women, Madness and English Culture 1830-1980*. Viarago Press: London.

Sibley, W. (1988), *Therapeutic Claims in Multiple Sclerosis*, Demos: NY

Sontag, S. (1988), *AIDS and Its Metaphors,* Harmondsworth: Penguin

Stacey, J. (1997), *A Cultural Study of Cancer*, London: Routledge.

Strauss, A; Corbin, J; Fagerhaugh, S; Glaser, B; Maines, D; Suczek, B and Wiener, C. (1984), *Chronic Illness and The Quality of Life*, The Mosby Company: USA (not in text)

Turner, B. S. (1992), *Regulating Bodies: Essays in Medical Sociology*, London: Routledge.

Ussher, J. (1991), *Women's Madness: Misogyny or Mental Illness?* Harvester Wheatsheaf: New York, London

Ussher, J. (1992), Reproductive rhetoric and blaming the body. In P. Nicolson and J. Ussher (Eds.) *The Psychology of Women's Health and Health Care* (pp. 31-61). London: Macmillan

Vanselow, W. (2000), What Does Systems Theory Have To Do With Premenstrual Complaints? In J. Ussher (Eds) *Womens' Health: Contemporary International Perspectives* (pp. 266-271) BPS Books: Leicester

In: Multiple Sclerosis Research Progress
Editors: H. Schwarz, L. Walter
ISBN: 978-1-60456-570-6
© 2008 Nova Science Publishers, Inc.

Chapter 8

NARRATIVE RESOURCES AND IDENTITY IN AN ONLINE SUPPORT GROUP FOR MULTIPLE SCLEROSIS

Monique Solomon

RESOURCEFULLY RESTORYING THE SELF ONLINE

Participation in an online support group is a social and personal act of resourcefully restorying the self. This chapter looks at how members of an online support group for Multiple Sclerosis (MS) draw upon medically and socially recognised discourses to present themselves as they story their experiences in spontaneous conversations on an online message board. In their posted messages, members invoke larger culturally available narrative resources and learn to engage the locally available narrative resources that emerge and develop from their online participation. Members actively and purposefully construct identity for those who will read their messages, as well as for themselves. Once posted, a message becomes a narrative record of the work of restorying the self. It can be reflected upon, responded to, rejected, challenged or embraced. The textual nature of online messages makes them important examples that reflect how individuals draw on narrative resources to accomplish identity online.

Although people with chronic illness are increasingly turning to the Internet for information and emotional support, "research exploring the development, use, and functions of illness-related groups online…remains limited" (Scheerhorn, 1997: 176). Few studies have addressed the relationship between grand narratives about illness and illness narratives "constructed by the afflicted themselves" (Hyden, 1997: 64). There have also been no comprehensive comparative studies regarding how illness narratives vary depending on the social context (Hyden, 1997). Studying online support groups speaks to the value of these groups as indicators of "how ideologies of health and illness reflect society's conflicting interests concerning disease prevention and the care of the sick" (Radley, 1994: 204). The online context affords a centralised position for observing and uncovering the socially valued narratives for talking about the self and illness. In this study, I address the relationship between social narratives and personal narratives and attend to narratives as they are storied by those who have chronic illness.

NARRATIVE, IDENTITY AND CHRONIC ILLNESS

Experiencing a chronic illness such as MS is a "call to restory the self" and rework identity not only in terms of the physical and embodied changes and challenges that accompany chronic illness but also in terms of social and cultural attitudes, values and beliefs surrounding illness (Frank, 1995). Chronic illness produces a change in social status. As Charmaz (1983: 168) contends, "chronically ill persons frequently experience a crumbling away of their former self-images without simultaneous development of equally valued new ones". Illness narratives hold the potential to rearticulate the illness experience and reconfigure social identity where the major disruptions produced by chronic illness have affected core components of identity, such as social roles and relationships (Hunt, 2000: 89).

In an effort to achieve a better understanding of how the experience of chronic illness is storied into our identity, we are encouraged to look at the whole story, analysing the structure and the content of a story as well as the available narrative resources that are drawn upon to create the story. By examining specific narrative texts online, we can recognise culturally relevant narrative resources drawn upon for accomplishing identity. Narrating experiences in terms of such things as social roles and relationships, and interpreting the "biographical disruption" (Williams, 2000) that results from chronic illness in terms of wider cultural narratives, reconstitutes identity (Riessman, 1990). Personal narratives are, thus, not only representations of experience but also active practices that help to socially construct experience and consequently help to restory the self as it is lived in the wider social and cultural world. In order to explore how identity is restoried in terms of chronic illness, this chapter considers together, the narrative resources available, and the artful activity used to story experience. In this way, we may consider how personal narratives engage with and integrate the contexts of larger discourse to accomplish identity.

RESEARCHING ONLINE SUPPORT GROUPS

The application of qualitative methodologies to the study of chronic illness aids in "exploring the subtleties and personal meanings that inhere to living with a chronic illness" (Conrad, 1990: 1257). Studies of online support groups indicate that they have a number of powerful and positive benefits. Online groups have been shown to have supportive benefits that align with "key life functions" of support as identified in face-to-face support groups including self care, mobilisation, communication, socialisation, employment (Braithwaite et al., 1999). Online support improves chances for outreach by addressing the social challenges of illness such as, living a restricted life, existing in social isolation, experiencing discredited definitions of self, and not wanting to become a burden to others (Charmaz, 1983). Further, it helps people with mobility-related challenges, or those who struggle with social and emotional challenges of face-to-face communication, to gain a sense of universality and community support while receiving information and learning from others (Braithwaite et al., 1999). As Conrad (1990: 1260) notes, "we need to study how people manage their illness in their everyday lives (for this) brings greater understanding to the specific illness and contributes to the general understanding of illness experience". By researching the social and personal narratives that members of an online group draw on to accomplish identity, we discover "opportunities for studying ongoing, everyday supportive interaction" (Braithwaite et al., 1999: 124).

Internet chat rooms and message boards provide a valuable site for studying illness narratives. They provide a contained, textual context that is conducive to studying narrative practices and everyday supportive interactions. Unlike traditional research in face-to-face support groups, members of online groups remain relatively anonymous to other members of the group and the researcher (see also Chapter 1 in this volume). The identity of members in the group is thoroughly composed in the choices they make about the content and format of their messages. Messages become mini-autobiographies that implicate a certain identity for the author. Here the self is thoroughly presented in a textual and narrative form that precludes other personal identifiers (that is, appearance, gestures, tone of voice).

By observing online message board postings, this study attends to illness narratives as they are practiced by "the afflicted themselves" (Hyden, 1997: 64). Rather than use an interview method involving formal questions between researcher and subject, this study concentrates on the conversational interactions between group members who share the common experience of having a chronic illness. This was decided based on the supposition that posing interview questions would change or influence the narrative style, and thus the types of narrative resources, that members of the group would drawn upon to talk about their experiences. The messages provided examples of conversational texts happening in real time and highlight the everyday narrative practices that characterise member's experiences of illness and the ways in which members draw on various narrative resources to accomplish identity.

METHOD

The Internet has become a key resource for gaining knowledge and support with regard to health and illness. Statistics Canada (2004) reported that in 2003 almost two-thirds (65%) of Canadian households had at least one member who used the Internet to search for medical or health-related information. Searching for health information on the Internet is now the third most popular use after e-mail and general browsing. For many people with chronic illness, the Internet is likely one of the first places to seek health information following diagnosis or the onset of symptoms. In choosing to explore sites that addressed chronic illness, I began by simply conducting an Internet search using a general search engine (www.google.ca/) just as someone who was newly diagnosed might look for a web site or information. Key words were "googled" to find support groups for chronic illnesses, for example, 'multiple sclerosis support groups'. The search generated thousands of web sites in a matter of seconds. Search parameters identified numerous online health and illness websites for chronic illnesses such as multiple sclerosis, cancer, HIV/AIDS, diabetes. To narrow down the possibilities, only the first few pages of listings were considered.

After a preliminary review of a number of possible sites, it became clear that selecting a site would not be as open as initially thought. According to online site disclaimers, many sites would not allow research or survey activity. Chat rooms and message boards that were sponsored or facilitated by medical organisations or pharmaceutical companies often included many pages of disclaimers. For example, one site listed thirteen message board guidelines including the following regarding online research: "The use of the message boards for gathering information for surveys and research studies is prohibited. You may inform people of a survey and invite them to participate by writing to you personally. Otherwise, these posts will be deleted." Disclaimers and restrictions of this kind speak to a broader discussion about the ethics of online research. According to Bakardjieva and Feenberg (2000: 233) "social life in cyberspace defies the existing procedures for obtaining informed consent from research subjects and groups". As the level and scope of online research continues to develop new ethical bodies are being set up to create guidelines for ethical conduct (Eysenbach, 2001).

While some sites were restrictive, web sites that were created, maintained and facilitated by independent individuals not affiliated with any organisation tended to be more open and welcoming. My personal interest and knowledge of multiple sclerosis led to the decision to focus on a web site for multiple sclerosis (MS). After considering a number of sites, one active online support group for people with MS and their families was selected. The site was founded and facilitated by someone with MS because, as she put it, she had "always worked and needed something to do…" and when asked she expressed surprise at the popularity of the site. At the time of the study the number of registered members in the group had reached 400 (see also Chapter 9 in this volume).

This MS web site offered both a real time chat room for group members and also an open public message board. To post a message on the board, it was necessary to join the group through a major chat room facilitator. However, posted messages could be accessed and read publicly without joining. In this study, care was taken to inform members of the researcher's intentions and the context of the research. With respect for the best interests of group members, full disclosure of the research was provided in an introductory online message posting to the group. The introductory message requested permission from online group members to conduct research regarding the stories and support they shared online. It also indicated that any information taken from the site would be made anonymous and messages that members wished not to be referenced would not be used.

Within twenty minutes of posting the Introductory Message, group members began responding with welcoming permission and encouragement. Once initial contact was made, I remained an observer in the group. I did not pose formal interview questions nor direct the online conversations. The intent of the study was to observe the spontaneous narratives taking place between group members who shared the experience of having MS. It is my supposition that the conversations and subsequent narrative practices shared between group members to story experiences would be influenced or impacted if formal questions were posed to the group.

Online observations took place over the course of two months (eight weeks) between November and January. The site was monitored daily. Posted messages were copied and saved in a word processing document, as they appeared online (i.e., text, grammar, pictures). Over the course of the eight weeks over 150 conversations were collected as posted on the message board. Messages were initially collected and reviewed by the date on which they appeared on the message board. They were sorted and reviewed according to the online titles given by the members (such as "Help with meds", "Newly diagnosed"). Online members who began a new conversational thread gave titles to their message board postings. The titles of the message postings served to inform group members of the topic, indicate the urgency of the message, and pique the interest of readers encouraging them to reply or respond.

Online Group Member's Responses to Introductory Script
Welcome. There are really great people here. I feel that the more people understand about this disease, the more they can support people touched by MS. Also, the greater the number of people who know about MS, the greater society's push will be for a cure. MONIQUE, GO FOR IT. THE MORE PUBLICITY THE BETTER FOR US. GOOD LUCK Monique, I think personally what you are doing is wonderful! I'll help anyway I can Take care and I hope you enjoy the site I don't know if my experience will help you at all, but if it does, you are more than welcome to use it. I hope this helps you Monique. I think what you are doing is great.

An initial review of the message postings provided an overall general impression of discursive characterisations and themes. Due to the larger volume of message board postings, a number of message samples were selected that best represented narrative resources that members called upon as they shared stories and support. The message samples in this chapter are presented as they appeared online (such as text, font style and so on) however, they have been edited for brevity, privacy and anonymity. Message samples for the project are discussed as they exemplify the prevalent discursive themes of the messages, the socially meaningful narrative resources used by members, and their implications for accomplishing identity.

Resourcefully Restoring the Self: Medical Talk, Social Meaning, Personal Expression, and Storying the Experience of Ms

Exploring how group members used narrative resources to accomplish their identities prompted consideration of what narrative themes and characterisations people call upon to convey who they are, as well as how narrative resources are practiced in their messages (Holstein and Gubrium, 2000). Holstein and Gubrium's (2000: 94) "analysis of interpretive practice" provided a methodological approach that allowed for flexibility to consider both *how* people tell stories about illness (practices) and *what* is involved in telling the story (narrative resources). The ability to take up the composition of the narrative and the discursive circumstances or contexts from which it is composed provided a unique perspective where we are invited to witness how the self is narratively accomplished. In other words, an analysis of interpretive practice offers a way to integrate how people talk about their experience of chronic illness, what culturally available narrative resources are implicated as they do so, and how these stories work to accomplish identity.

Analytic bracketing does not hold narrative practices or the resources that inform them as a standard discursive reality. Rather, it allows for a deliberation of the active interplay between personal and cultural narratives of illness. It alternately contemplates how people share experiences of illness narratives with what structures and contexts are implicated as they are expressed. Narratives are seen to be experientially real and are taken for what they represent in the moment, for those who are doing the narrating. Employing Holstein and Gubrium's (2000: 95) method of "analytic bracketing" does not aim to limit or define the ways that we talk about illness. It requires us to concentrate on the discursive interplay between resources and construction thus allowing us to glimpse the narrative possibilities for accomplishing identity. In the analysis for this study, online message samples are presented and discussed as they relate to four identifiable thematic narrative resources emerging from the data: medical talk, social meanings, personal expression, and storying the experience of MS.

Medical Talk: Diagnosis, Symptoms, Treatment

The majority of the messages posted by members of the online group exemplified how readily medical discourse has been taken up to accomplish identity. Discussions of diagnosis, symptoms and treatments were the most prevalent narrative resources drawn upon. Members of the online group authenticated membership – and identity – in the group as someone diagnosed, waiting to be diagnosed, or not yet diagnosed. Messages reflected unique experiential understandings of the diagnostic process, the symptoms attributed to MS, and the treatments available. Members sought or offered advice based on narrative resources provided by medical discourse but in doing so transposed the information in a way that made it personal and individual.

About Multiple Sclerosis (MS)

In order to contextualise the narratives presented in this study it is important to provide some background information about the illness that members in the online group are experiencing.

- MS is the most common neurological disease affecting young adults in Canada.
- MS can cause loss of balance, impaired speech, extreme fatigue, double vision and paralysis.
- Canadians have one of the highest rates of multiple sclerosis in the world.
- Every day, three more people in Canada are diagnosed with MS.
- MS was first identified and described by a French neurologist, Dr. Jean-Martin Charcot, in 1868.
- We don't know what causes MS but researchers are closer to finding the answer.

Source: MS Society of Canada *http://www.mssociety.ca/en/information/default.htm*

Diagnosis

Multiple Sclerosis (MS) does not generally come upon people suddenly. Individuals may experience several years of physical discomfort, temporary bouts with disability, or a gradual decline in ability before ever seeking medical advice. The action of seeking medical advice is different for everyone. Generally speaking, it is only when physical discomforts or abilities become severe or do not diminish that a person seeks advice from medical and other health professionals. In some cases, this leads to a quick and clear definition, while in other cases, the 'relief' of having a diagnosis – of giving a name to what ails us – is elusive and frustrating. Faith in the experts to provide an answer often becomes a key focus. Once a diagnosis is made, the reality of this new label prompts a re-evaluation of identity -- a need to restory the self in terms of the medical definition while at the same time retaining a sense of pre-diagnosis identity, integrating new symptomatic descriptions and learning to incorporate new terminology to describe the self.

For members of the online group, diagnosis was a powerful narrative resource for accomplishing identity. Members presented themselves in terms of being diagnosed, not diagnosed, not yet diagnosed, or waiting to be diagnosed. Members most often provided this information in their first time postings (for example, even in my own introductory message posting, I inadvertently identified myself as "not having been diagnosed"). In response to first time postings long-time members responded by providing information about their own diagnosis as a way of welcoming a new member.

Diagnosis

i'm... my nickname is really... i was diagnosed in oct. 2000. i had been having problems for a couple of years before that. i remember thinking i was really out of shape and that if i excercised more my legs would stop feeling so weak. boy was i wrong on that one!! the more i excercised the shakier my legs got. then i decided that i couldn't walk without feeling unbalanced because i was anemic or something. wrong again!! one night while sitting on the couch it felt like one of my kids was dropping cold water on my feet. the kids were no where around. when i told my doctor she decided to do an mri and the rest is history.

Hi... i was dx nov.2000 as of last year... ...like you for years i could not figure out what was wrong with me i never went to see a doctor until my left leg became parylyzed at first i ended up in the emergency room.luckily i was dx right away my neuro said my first outward sign was when i had optic neuritis... ...when i got my dx it sure did answer a lot of questions about how i was feeling for years.i suppose i should have gone to see a doctor sooner but i did not know how to describe what was going on with my body i figured they would think i was nuts !! 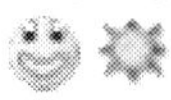

I still haven't received a diagnosis **yet**! ...My two Neurologists (Tweedle Dumb and Tweedle Dumber) still don't know what is wrong. ...(test) showed clear so Dumb said no MS even though I have sevaral lesions..., he said symptoms mean nothing; alot of people have symptoms.

That is good news you can all stop your meds!! You just have symptoms and not MS!!

...All I want is a diagnosis and I can't get one because nothing is wrong. I guess; that's what I'll have on my tombstone - "there was something wrong but we don't know what." I lost my mind but not my humor. When I lose that you'll know it's really bad. ...my friend called yesterday and his brother has Parkinsons and it took 18 years to diagnose; maybe there **is** hope for me! I only have to wait 17 more years; I am sure it will fly by.

In the first message, sample group members introduce themselves using narrative resources referring to family roles as well as their experiences of 'getting a diagnosis'. In the final message posting shown here, a member expresses frustration at waiting for a diagnosis. Calling upon narratives resources that value the education and experience of medical professionals, the member personally draws on other narratives resources; in this case literary, taken from a children's story to describe her experience with some sarcasm and humour[1]. The importance of a timely diagnosis also evidenced by the reference made to a friend's brother's experience with a diagnosis of Parkinson's. Being diagnosed provides credibility to members' stories giving them a sense of permission to begin restorying themselves as someone with MS. As this member awaits a diagnosis, there is uncertainty with regard to symptoms and identity.

Diagnosis as someone with MS becomes a way of presenting an authentic identity that meets the local culture of the group. It positions a member within the group by defining their experiences in terms of the available narrative resources provided by medical discourse. Certainly, the process of diagnosis and the experiences of being diagnosed are different for all members of the group but being able to name the outcome of those experiences in one way – multiple sclerosis – is an important step in accomplishing identity.

Symptoms

MS is most commonly described as a disease where the symptoms are different for everyone; however, medical discourse provides common symptom terminology for MS. Members in the group were skilled at talking about symptoms in medical terms and integrating these terms into personal narratives. The online support group provided a place to discover if a member's symptoms were representative of having MS. In message postings about symptoms, members often asked others for clarification about symptoms they were experiencing.

As the sample indicates, members creatively develop and share a special terminology for certain symptoms that are specific to MS. In requesting information about a "tightness and numbing feeling in the upper body", a member discovers that not only is this symptom a common one but it has been given special names by those who experience it -- "MS Hug" or "the girdle effect". This provides a local narrative resource that helps members define themselves as someone who has MS. In this way, identity is actively constructed as members

[1] "Tweedle Dumb and Tweedle Dumber" refers to two dimwitted characters (Tweedledum and Tweedledee) in the classic tale, Alice's Adventures in Wonderland by Lewis Carroll (1865).

position their experiences in terms of personal narrative resources provided by others. Members responding to the initial request often confirm a similar experience making this a symptom that members may call upon to identify with having MS.

Symptoms
Does anyone have a problem with tightness and numbing in there upper body.It not painful just annoying. Yes! Honey! It's called the "MS Hug" and can stay with you for a while but WILL go away! I thought it was my bra or tight clothes or just plain fat! However, once you know what the cause is, the problem seems less stressful. Hope all goes OK with you! LOL! I've heard it called "the girdle" effect. I get it all the time from one side of my stomache to the other. I also have the "tightness" around my chest too, but that could be from other things… or just plain getting old and shrinking! LOL

Treatments

Medical research into treatments for MS are abundant and learning about treatment availability, side effects, and treatment efficacy were popular topics of discussion in the online group studied here.[2] Although Internet sites for pharmaceutical companies and other medical or health sites provide volumes of information about MS treatments, membership in the online group offers an experiential and individual perspective. Members learn the medical terminology of treatments and then take up this language to restory their experiences in personal ways when talking with others. Identifying oneself as knowledgeable and experienced with certain treatments further solidifies group membership and identity as someone with MS. As medical research continues to offer up new and improved versions of numerous pharmaceutical treatments for MS, members create their own local jargon for talking about treatment options often abbreviating the most predominant treatment choices by referring to them as the ABCRs (Avonex, Betaseron, Copaxone, Rebif).

In this message sample, members work diligently to share their experiences with the "ABCRs" and in doing so draw on a number of narrative resources to story their identities. Messages include references to significant social relationships, career, and physical and psychological experiences (for example, mom, spouse, employee, informed consumer, depression).

---

[2] Message postings regarding medical and pharmaceutical treatments were significantly more common although in a few cases members briefly discussed complementary and alternative treatments (e.g., massage, tai chi).

Treatments

Hi everyone! I need a little help making up my mind. I went back to the neuro and he felt that it was time for me to choose one of the ABC's. I have narrowed it down to Copaxone or Avonex. I have gone to the individual drug websites, looked in some drug books to get information about them. Now I thought it might be good to ask those of you who are on or have been on either one of these your thoughts. I know that results/experiences may vary. I am a young mom with two kids... I work part time... my spouse is not always home to help out... I have alot of depressing coplications... ...I didn't list my life elements not to whine, but to maybe help you to give your point of view and advise. ...

I have been on Copaxone for just over a year now. 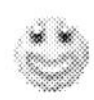 Things have got better and the daily jab is so small it's not worth worrying about. I was told it takes 6 months to start working and I would go along with that. People say the jab does nothing to you but I feel it has and would recommend it to anyone. Good luck with your choice Be as well as you can be

Do you have a problem with Interferons? I do. So I have to take Copaxone. When you are first starting out on the ABCR's you just make your best educated guess and go with it. You can always change. Of course I listened to everyone else about the flu symptoms of A for months before I decided that no drug was better than being sick with the flu ALL the time. I was on C for X years and progressed downward, so I tried B for X weeks and had a major set backs. So I went back to C. Yes you do need to take a drug because there is nothing else to offer at this point but trial and error is the only method that works in picking which one.

I was on Betasaron for X yrs. Had a major attack, lost my job and my insurance and Beta would not work with me for financial help. I had the flu like symptoms for the first X months.

I was on nothing for X months until Avonex approved to help. I love the once a week injection verses the every other day with Beta. ...I have had no side effects from Avonex at all. Personally, I don't want to inject myself daily, as you would with Cop, but each person has diff needs and you will have to decide what works best for you.

Members identify themselves by stating which treatment they are on or have tried and why. And members present themselves as educated about the treatments from an experiential and individual standpoint. This leads to a restorying of self in terms of treatment experiences. Identity is accomplished with reference to treatment names and options chosen – "I chose Avonex" or "I have been on Copaxone". As well, the self is storied in light of personal experience – "things have got better" or "I had flu-like symptoms". Members encourage each other to "do what works best for you" and comment that making a choice is a "personal preference". These comments inform personal narratives that support individuality in treatment choices and yet positions identity in terms of what treatments are being used.

Social Meaning: Relationships and Roles

Whereas narrative resources provided by medical discourses contributed to how illness was storied by providing specific discursive guidelines concerning diagnosis, symptoms and treatments, it is the integration of a variety of socially meaningful narrative resources outside of medical talk that offer personal depth and meaning to illness narratives. Socially constructed through the discursive forces that prevail and predominate in our culture, social meanings of illness express more than just the physical manifestations of disease. They express the social, economic, and political realities of living with illness. How we come to talk about and *do* illness is closely intertwined with other social and cultural discourses in an artful and individual way. It is an "interpretive salvage operation" in which selves are "craft(ed) from the vast array of available resources" (Holstein and Gubrium, 2000: 153).

Invoking culturally relevant and available resources that have personal meaning, members more comfortably and successfully restory their experiences and their identity online. Many message postings contained what Holstein and Gubrium (2000: 169) call "biographical particulars". In narrating a story about the everyday going concerns of having illness, members often included socially relevant biographical particulars and effectively presented themselves in reference to their careers, marital status, and other life experiences. In doing so, members were "engaged in ordinary 'biographical work' to assemble aspects of personal history that can be used to bolster claims of and about themselves" (Holstein and Gubrium, 2000:169). The value of these claims is that they provide a wider context for the self that emerges from understood social values and narratives.

Relationships

It was evident from the majority of message postings that members do not experience illness in a socially isolated world. Relationships play a vital role in the social experience of illness giving it social and personal meaning. A powerful and long time cultural discourse in our society is one in which a person with illness is supported and aided by family members. We see in the next sample posting how group members draw on socially significant narrative resources about family and parenthood to resourcefully present the challenges that illness and social role expectations bring.

Here members draw on culturally available narrative resources about what it means to be a good parent while implicating narrative resources about taking responsibility for self. In this message, members integrate social narratives about parenthood and expectations of children and family to negotiate what it means to be a responsible parent with MS. There is a struggle to incorporate the idea that 'family should help family' in the case of illness, yet as a parent the first priority is still an expectation of caring for their children. Members share biographical particulars of parenthood to story identities first as parents and then as parents with MS. Identifying as parents they express a desire to be there for their children but in their experience with MS they draw on narratives about family helping family and that it is okay to ask for support. As one member stated, "...In all reality though it is really our family and friends that we do need to reach out to in our time of need".

Relationships
I know it was my fault I didn't take my cane This is going to sound stupid, but I decided to walk home from my (grown child's) house. It started raining and I was getting soaked…It is not that far, but I should have know better …I fell in the door coming in. (My spouse) thought I had got a ride home. … they didn't have much gas so I didn't want to ask… … I was just trying to save (them) from…wasting gas. …I just don't wan't to be a burden to people. That is why I didn't even want to ask for a ride…. I know where your coming from.My hubby …feels that there are no excuses for certain ways that the kids are or hwo they are.I am from the old school also but i know if it was my mom nomatter what she would have been in my car and she would not have to ask me there would have been no 2 ways about it. We should not excuse our kids for not doing because that in my opinion makes them feel that nothing else matters more then their needs. … What i am trying to say is to you and everyone else is we do need some special help from time to time and our loved ones that we ourselves would bend over backwords for should help.When we were all in better shape i am sure that most of us did plenty … … A ride home ---- a phone call-------a trip to a store etc should not be a burden for people who we love and love us!!!! …i know how you feel. i have X kids… … my…son is great. he helps me and dad all the time. when he gets up in the morning he asks what we need him to do today. the X-year old is very understanding, too. when we have problems doing things he always says "it's just part of living with ms." it's really cute. the others often make me feel like dad and i got ms just so we could inconvenience them. hang in there and next time on the *ride* home don't forget your cane…. …i am so sorry to hear about what happened to you how inconsiderate of your (grown child) …you need to start thinking about what you can do or cant do and speak up for your self and say NO i cant do that! … i never leave my house with out my cane even for a very short distance, i am sure that you will always be taking your cane along

Roles

Although there are many ways to think about being a productive member of society the prevalent concerns expressed by members of the online group also focused greatly on careers and employability.

Roles
... I work filltime ...Since my diagnosis ... Ive missed a great deal of work - ...with each attack depending on the severity and symptoms as it all affects my ability to work and be productive. My employer is VERY understanding and encourages me to stay home as long as I need to get better. ...but I always rush back to work (trying to be as normal as possible) only to get sick again...I am now off once again...I feel soooo guilty not being there. Is there anyone in the same boat as me or have most people out there taken time for themselves to get better 'fully' before going back to work. ... If I ever lost my job Id be crushed.....Any advice or people in simliar situations? I am having guilt problems too. Though I have worked through most of my attacks... since I dont have a Definate DX, I cannot justify missing a lot of work. ... THere is not a whole lot I can do, I have to work for the insurance and without a DX i cannot get the meds and without the Dx I cannot get disability. I would have to say if your empolyer encourages you to stay off work until you are better take full advantage of their encouragement. ... I was not as fortunate as you, I was working ...when I had my first bad attack I was off work for about X months. ... Before my neurologist could even type up my diagnosis my employer terminated me ...there was alot of discrimination issues, my boss had the nerve to ask me to my face "What happens if you have another attack later on down the road, are we suppose to accomidate you by letting you take off work?"

Expressions of guilt, anxiety, and concern over not being able to work are further underscored by social realities that have not yet created space for alternative working lifestyles such as those that may be required in the case of chronic illness. Here members story their identity in terms of their employment experiences indicating just how prevalent and powerful this social narrative resource is as an indicator of identity.

Personal Expression

The ability to communicate online can be both liberating and limited. For those who have found this virtual space to share support and stories, it is a haven for expressing doubts, fears, and concerns about having a chronic illness. It is also a place to commiserate and celebrate with others who share similar experiences. Online support lacks the usual visual cues that expressions of support entail (such as eye contact, gestures, touch, tone of voice). With no "scenic presence" (Holstein and Gubrium, 2000: 190), online members do not share social spaces nor see or hear each other in person so there is more reliance on textual and visual cues to relate personal expressions and in essence personality and identity.

In the message samples reviewed in this study, it was pleasantly evident that there was more to posting a message than just the text. Members used different fonts and colours, and included emotional signifiers (emoticons), pictures, special online names, and positive sign-offs ("Be as well as you can be"), thereby, presenting a unique identity online. Holstein and Gubrium (2000, p. 187) draw our attention to these "material mediations" for storying the self, suggesting that the stories we construct are mediated by our material environment, social settings and the physical cues around us. The online support group is a unique example of this.

The addition of a smiley face  or a sad face  within the messages expressed the emotions of the person, or indicated their view on a discussion providing insight about a member's opinions and beliefs. Pictures used in messages provided metaphoric social and cultural resources that communicated information about identity (like lone wolf). By adding visual characterisations, members include a sense of individuality and emotion in their messages. Even in the simplest textual messages presented online, we gain a sense of who a person is by how they construct and present their messages. Restricted by the material mediations online, members endeavoured to assemble available materials in their own unique ways adding personal expression and identity cues to their messages.

The sample box below displays some of the visual resources (emoticons, pictures) used by members in their message postings. Other unique characteristics that members used to convey personal expressions included different styles and colours of text. Special care was taken to preserve the message samples throughout these results as they appeared online. However, to preserve confidentiality, special online names and sign-off messages have been omitted from the message samples.

Personal Expression

Emoticons

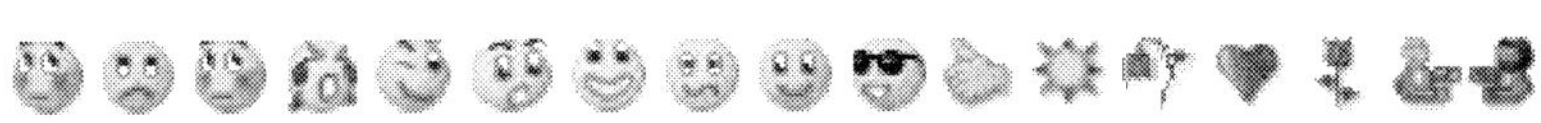

Pictures

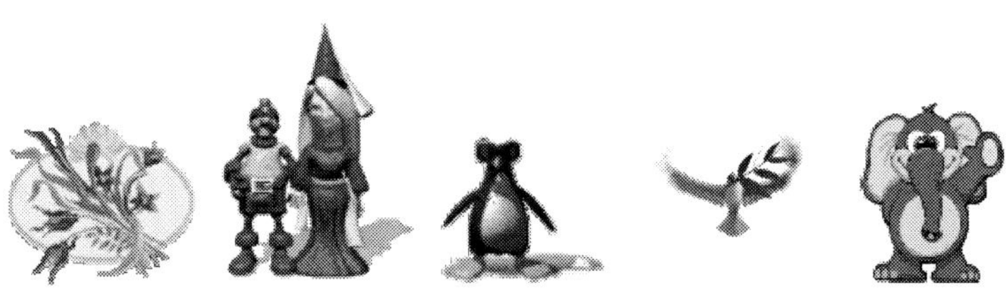

Storying the Experience of MS: Supporting Others, Being Positive

"People tell stories not just to work out their own changing identities, but also to guide others who will follow them" (Frank, 1995: 17). In a final analysis of the message postings, it was evident that members in the group were routinely generous with encouragement, appreciation, and support. Referencing their personal experiences with MS, members acknowledged difficulties but did so in a positive and supportive manner. There was little talk of "why me?" and more talk about facing adversity and being "as well as you can be". Members used humour and enthusiasm in their messages. Message postings that were seen as rude, negative, or of a commercial nature were quickly deleted. Local group "conventions and constraints" evidently required members to remain positive, supportive and on topic (Holstein and Gubrium, 2000: 182).

Two predominant local narratives for storying the experience of MS emerged from the data -- supporting others and being positive. These two ways of storying the experience of MS are characteristic of almost every message posted during the study. The prevalence of this way of talking about illness experiences indicates the power and significance of this narrative resource for storying experiences and identity as someone with MS.

Supporting Others

Group members regularly identified themselves as supportive and productive members in their online and real life MS communities. Taking up this supportive role indicated an authentic position as someone with MS. It was a key signifier of acceptance into a community and identity as someone with MS. The founder of the online group expresses the value and importance she placed on helping others.

Supporting Others

What made me start this site is that I realized that is that I knew that I was not alone in dealing with MS. I would start a site and even if only 1 person joined, that made it worth it.

Did I expect to get over 400 ? Not in my Dreams
Also, I have always worked and I needed something to do.

In response to a message of distress, online members provided the following messages of support…

I know (from your post) that you are going through a hard time, but things will be looking up! If it's prayer you want, prayer you will get! There are many members here that are close to God and I'm sure we'll all put in a prayer for you. Even those that aren't religious will probably have some nice thoughts and well wishes.

If you ever need a shoulder to lean on I am here. If you would like you can e-mail me at… I realize that in this situation there is so much stress and that alone is bad for the MS. …

…Just to let you know you arent the only person out there dealing with these same problems. I think if you could share with us a little more detail about your situation you would find that some of us are going through the same things that you are and we might actually be able to help each other out. Be strong things will work out. This is

the best place to come for comfort and support and just to vent....
We all understand how you feel as we are all fighting daily battles, fears, and doubts. This is the best place to come where we can share our joys and sadness and others can relate to. ... Remember we are all here to help each other... you have our positive thoughts and we all wish you the strength to face each day knowing you are not alone.

Members continually posted messages of support for others that worked to confirm their authentic position in the group via their own personal understandings of having MS. In the sample above members draw on a number of socially meaningful narrative resources and local group narratives thereby accomplishing their identity online (such as religion, spiritually, strength by virtue of group membership and similar life experiences, value of sharing emotional distress).

Being Positive

Being positive and hopeful are key narratives for storying identity as someone with MS. From brief words of encouragement, i.e.,"good luck", "be well", to longer messages of support and guidance, members of the group actively and continuously storied their experiences in terms of being positive. The "be positive" narrative appeared in some form in almost every message posted during the study. The final message samples were taken from a variety of available message postings. The samples indicate the sincerity and value that this group placed on this local narrative resource and suggest just how important this way of storying the experience of MS is for accomplishing identity in the group.

Being Positive
... Our physical difficulties are circumstances that we cannot control but our mental circumstances are a choice for most of us. We can choose to be depressed and sad or we can choose to make the best of it and do the best that we can. When we are truly doing the best that we can, we cannot do more than that. If one thinks about that for a minute it should give some peace. When one is at point such as this the only acceptable choice is to make the best of it. Don't ask "why me" because there is no answer. It is frustrating to ask a question that has no answer so don't bother with the question. This may sound simple and that is because it is simple. It is a simple choice, your choice.
MS... i always remind myself i definatly could be worse (will I is Question that I can't answer and try never to harp on at all). I do not resent that I have MS because I am a person who feels instead of why me? ,I say to myself why NOT me.Why someone else and not me. ...we have to go on and make the best of each day we can. ...I though am extreamly grateful for days that I feel good.

> … the human spirit that is in all of us can overcome any obstacle… MS is a problem for sure but it isn't anything that we can't handle. Since being diagnosed one of the most rewarding experiences of my life is helping others with ms. Never in my wildest dreams did I ever expect this to be the case but it is. MS has not been a negative influence on my life. I guess it was in the beginning but for the past X yrs. or so it has been like a good teacher. Some of the lessons are hard but you really learn things that otherwise might have passed you by. …

As the sample excerpts indicate, narrative resources for doing chronic illness guide members to "do the best you can", "find alternatives", "don't ask why me". These gentle directives inform members of the importance of staying positive and persevering. And because they appear so often, they become a guide for the group and for others to recognise that living with chronic illness takes strength, character and a positive attitude. Just as medical discourse provides certain narrative resources, i.e.,diagnosis, symptoms, for talking about chronic illness which help to define identity (e.g., I have MS); the way that members talk about personal experiences of illness ("we have a choice", "do the best you can") guides others to story the self in locally appropriate ways (i.e.,positive, persevering).

A Narrative Map for Chronic Illness

This study takes up a central position between narrative resources and narrative practices -- one providing the building blocks for constructing identity and the other providing an active and discursive space for assembling and practicing how the self is storied everyday. At this theoretical intersection, we have examined the characteristic options that are available for people with chronic illness to accomplish identity. Attending to how members narratively construct and negotiate messages online affords us the ability to discern what the most prevalent narrative options for storying the self might be.

The analysis of the study suggests that there is a pattern for how members of the online support group draw on narrative resources to story their experiences and accomplish their identity online. The prevalence with which some narrative resources are drawn upon by members of the online group suggests that there is a "narrative map" that frames and guides how to talk about chronic illness, in this case multiple sclerosis (Frank, 1995; Pollner and Stein, 1996). This narrative map is not a formal template. It is an informal guide for members of the group to negotiate, draw upon, and contribute to as they come to accomplish identity as someone with chronic illness.

New members come to the group seeking ways to story their experiences when the general ways of talking about their physical discomforts and limited abilities no longer fit. Members of the online group studied here framed and expressed their experiences online in terms of medical talk about diagnosis, symptoms and treatments. These became the pervasive ways of talking about both experiences of MS and the self. Learning the narrative languages of other discourse communities (such as medical) members integrated this language into their own narratives of illness. Members also incorporated socially meaningful narrative resources to story their identity using biographical particulars (that is being a parent, employment). They incorporated the changes that illness brings into other socially meaningful ways of talking about experiences and self. The great number of references to social relationships indicates that this is a significant element of the narrative map for chronic illness.

Over time members became increasingly knowledgeable about the specific discursive frameworks for storying the illness experiences that characterise MS (that is being positive, supporting others). Members of the group drew on social and medical narrative resources and were actively engaged in practicing and producing their own personal narrative resources, guiding others about how to talk about MS. Through this active dialogue and interaction with others the narrative resources were reified, challenged, embraced and made richer from the addition of member's personal experiences. They were refined and developed as they were resourcefully practiced and shared by members of the group. All of the narrative resources became part of a dynamic online repertoire for talking about the experience of MS.

Conclusion: A Resourcefully Practiced Self

The work of restorying the self is a complex and exhausting process. To hold down and essentialise the self in terms of personality traits or inherently individual characteristics loses sight of the active, variable, and continuous possibilities for discursively accomplishing identity. Faced with an excess of possible narrative resources and a multitude of sites for narrative practice, members of online support groups for chronic illness frame their experiences and identity in terms of the narrative resources accessible to them in everyday interactions. Online support groups offer people with chronic illness an opportunity to actively engage in restorying the self by drawing on personal and social narrative resources. Group members are guided by these narrative resources and map out an authentic and acceptable identity for others and for themselves. The self is resourcefully practised.

In this chapter, we considered how drawing from a shared pool of available narrative resources (for example, medical, social, personal), members of the online group actively work to interpret and express themselves in light of their personal experience. A negotiation and translation of sorts occurs as members share personal experiences with others using different styles, characteristics and choices of expression (that is emoticons, special names, attitudes, beliefs). As Holstein and Gubrium (2000: 11) suggest, "self-interpretation involves social input to be sure, but it's also a matter of interpretive practice, of putting forth the effort and engaging in the everyday work of orienting to each other as selves". In the sample messages, personal experience is seen to work as both a resource and a filter for engagement with available narrative resources. By expressing and interpreting available resources in individual ways a self is presented that is at once "practical, variegated, and artfully and deliberately built up in various shapes and dimensions for dealing with the circumstances in which it is located" (Holstein and Gubrium, 2000: 10).

Attending to illness narratives opens up discursive space for exploring the narrative resources that are drawn upon to story the experience of chronic illness. In online message postings, the illness experience is textually crafted into something uniquely individual and yet it holds to socially accepted narrative structures and those essentialised by local group narratives. Taken as a whole, the online messages indicate patterns or narrative maps for how to do illness. Reflecting on how these narrative maps are practiced and shared in everyday interactions, we gain a more nuanced understanding of the experience of chronic illness and the discursive moves that are implicated as members share stories and support to accomplish identity online.

ACKNOWLEDGMENTS

Special thanks to the members of the MS online support group whose stories appear in this chapter.

REFERENCES

Bakardjieva, M. and Feenberg, A., 2001, 'Involving the Virtual Subject: Conceptual, Methodological and Ethical Dimensions' *Journal of Ethics and Information Technology*, vol. 2, no. 4, pp. 233-240.

Braithwaite, D. O., Waldron, V. R. and Finn, J, 1999, 'Communication of Social Support in Computer-Mediated Groups for People With Disabilities', *Health Communication*, vol. 11, no. 2, pp. 123-151.

Charmaz, K., 1983, 'Loss of Self: A Fundamental Form of Suffering in the Chronically Ill', *Sociology of Health & Illness*, Vol. 5, no. 2, pp. 168-195.

Conrad, P., 1990, 'Qualitative Research on Chronic Illness: A Commentary on Method and Conceptual Development', *Social Science & Medicine*, vol. 30, no. 11, pp. 1257-1263.

Eysenbach, G. and Till, J. E., 2001, 'Information in Practice: Ethical Issues in Qualitative Research on Internet Communities', *British Medical Journal. <http://bmj.bmjjournals.com/cgi/content/full/323/7321/1103>*

Frank, A. W., 1995, *The Wounded Storyteller: Body, Illness, and Ethics*, The University of Chicago Press, Chicago.

Holstein, J. A. and Gubrium, J. F., 2000, *The Self We Live By: Narrative Identity in a Postmodern World*, Oxford University Press, New York.

Hunt, L. M., 2000, 'Strategic Suffering: Illness Narratives as Social Empowerment Among Mexican Cancer Patients', in C. Mattingly and L. C. Garro (eds.), *Narrative and the Cultural Construction of Illness and Healing*, pp. 88-107, University of California Press, Berkeley.

Hyden, L.C., 1997, 'Illness and Narrative', *Sociology of Health & Illness*, vol. 19, no. 1, pp. 48-69.

Pollner, M. and Stein, J., 1996, 'Narrative Mapping of Social Worlds: The Voice of Experience in Alcoholics Anonymous', *Symbolic Interaction*, vol. 19, no. 3, pp. 203-233.

Radley, A., 1994, *Making Sense of Illness*, Sage Publications, London.

Reissman, C. K.,1990, 'Strategic Uses of Narrative in the Presentation of Self and Illness: A Research Note', *Social Science & Medicine*, vol. 30, no. 11, pp. 1195-1200.

Scheerhorn, D, 1997, 'Creating Illness-Related Communities in Cyberspace', in J. Richard, L. Street, W. R. Gold and T. Manning (eds.), *Health Promotion and Interactive Technology: Theoretical Applications and Future Directions*, pp. 171-185, Lawrence Erlbaum Associates Publishers, Mahwah, New Jersey.

Statistics Canada, 2004, 'Household Internet Use Survey. Science, Innovation and Electronic Information Division'.<*http://www.statcan.ca/Daily/English/040708/d04070 8a.htm*>

Williams, S. J., 2000, 'Chronic Illness as Biographical Disruption or Biographical Disruption as Chronic Illness? Reflections on a Core Concept', *Sociology of Health & Illness*, vol. 22, no. 1, pp. 40-67.

In: Multiple Sclerosis Research Progress
Editors: H. Schwarz, L. Walter
ISBN: 978-1-60456-570-6
© 2008 Nova Science Publishers, Inc.

Chapter 9

COGNITIVE IMPAIRMENTS IN MULTIPLE SCLEROSIS

Katarzyna Prochwicz[1], Anna Starowicz[2] and Janusz Otfinowski[2]
[1]Psychology Department, Jagiellonian University, Krakow, Poland
[2]Rehabilitation Department, Collegium Medicum Jagiellonian University, Krakow, Poland

ABSTRACT

The changes in emotional and cognitive functioning of patients with MS can be divided into two groups. The first one consists of psychological changes being patients' adaptive reactions to their illness like exogenous depression, neurotic reactions and hypochodrical syndromes. In the second group there are changes caused by the demyelination process (brain damage), for instance, dysfunctions of cognitive and intellectual sphere, and psychiatric syndromes (depression, emotional lability, and uncontrolled crying and laughter). The article focuses on the latter and offers a review of the latest research results on cognitive disorders in multiple sclerosis.

In the beginning we present specific cognitive disorders resulting from damages in particular brain locations as well as unspecific cognitive problems caused by the scattered brain damages. Speech impairments, especially dysarrthria, are described most carefully. Moreover, the article provides a report on recent data showing that MS patients suffer also from long and short- term memory impairments and difficulties in learning the new material.

The article contains the characteristics of dementia in the course of MS.
Then we discuss the complex relations among four elements: intensity of neurological dysfunctions, clinical course of the multiple sclerosis, its type, and the characteristics of cognitive impairments.

The last part of the article contains a review of the research on the role of neuropsychological tasks and computer programs designed to support the MS patients in their rehabilitiation process aimed to improve their cognitive functioning and prevent, or at least slow down, the further negative changes in this area.

Multiple sclerosis (MS) is a chronic, neurological disease that destroys the myelin sheath and creates demyelinated lesions (plaques) which are situated mainly in the brain white substance and rarely in the cerebral cortex. In most cases plaques are located in the lateral ventricles of the brain, sometimes subcortically in the frontal and parietal area, hardly ever in the occipital, temporal, thalamus and commissura magna lobes.The demyelination process may vary in intensity, from singular occurrence of demyelinated axons up to vast demyelination with inflammatory infiltrations around blood vessels and edema (Szepietowska: 1997). The damage of axons due to demyelination lesions leads to progressive motor disabilities, peripheral dysesthesia, acroparesthesia and paresthesia of the trunk and head. In later stages of the disease hypertonia occurs, especially attacking higher and lower limbs with muscular contractures hindering movement.

Clinical Overview of MS Cognitive Impairments

Mental disorders occurring among patients with multiple sclerosis may be divided into two groups of sensations. The first one consists of adjustment reactions' symptoms which are the consequences of the development of the illness and the fact of patients experiencing it as a critical state. The second group consists of cognitive and emotional symptoms being a direct result of changes happening in the nervous system. Publications regarding MS, besides the neurological symptoms connected with motor and emotional functioning, more and more often describe the cognitive deficiencies resulting from demyelination processes, which fit into the second group of the aforementioned mental disorders. These studies focus upon the description of cognitive impairments characteristic for MS, taking into consideration the influence of such factors as course and duration of the disease, extent of motor disability and pharmacological treatment (Szepietowska: 1997). Some of the publications also attempt to describe the relationship between cognitive impairments and the extent and localization of demyelination lesions in the central nervous system (e.g., Arnett et al.: 1994; Rao et al.: 1991; Swirsky-Sacchetti et al.: 1992), as well as to determine the influence of fatigability and mood disorders on the development and intensification of these symptoms (Bruce, Arnett: 2004; Feinstein: 2006; Parmenter, Dougals, Lynch: 2003).

The MS cognitive impairments, which are the most frequently illustrated, are memory, attention and speech, abstract thinking and executive functions impairments. Simultaneously the publications emphasize the huge diversity of results gathered from neuropsychological tests done by patients and of the problems caused by this fact in formulating general and definite conclusions concerning MS cognitive functioning impairments (Feinstein: 2004).

Memory Disorders

The most frequent symptoms of cognitive impairments among MS patients are problems regarding memory. Memory disorders were observed in 40-60% of MS cases (Brassington, Marsch: 1998). Former research on MS memory disorders concentrated on three main topics:

1. Functioning of short-term memory and disorders regarding consolidation of memory trace.
2. Disorders of recalling the information from long-term memory.
3. Deficiencies in information organizing strategies during the stage of learning and remembering, resulting from metamemory disorders.

Research on functioning of short-term memory among MS patients has not brought straightforward outcomes. Most of the results indicate that functioning of short-term memory reveals no trace of any disorder or is subjected to only slight disturbances (Heaton, Nelson, Thompson: 1985; Rao, Hammeke, Mc Quilen: 1984; Ron, Callanan: 1991). However, there has been some research conducted among MS patients proving their problems with consolidation of memory trace, intensifying through introduction of a distracter between a situation involving learning and one involving remembering. This fact illustrates a small increase in memorizing efficiency of information repeated in consecutive turns (Grant, Mc Donald, Trimble, 1984) and low efficiency in recalling a list of words, especially in circumstances which do not allow quiet repeating of information during their exposure (Beatty et al.: 1988; Caine et al.: 1986; Rao, Hammerke, Speech: 1987; Van der Burg, Van Zomeren: 1987).

A more coherent spectrum of symptoms was achieved in case of long-term memory disorders. Much research indicates explicit deficiencies in this area of study among MS patients (Beatty, Gange: 1977; Beatty et al.: 1988; Fisher: 1988; Heaton et al.: 1985; Minden et al.: 1990; Rao et al.: 1984). Most of the authors combine the origin of memory impairments in MS patients with their difficulties in evoking information from long-term memory, in spite of well-preserved coding and memory trace consolidation abilities (Caine et al.: 1986; Grafman et al.: 1990; Rao: 1993). This opinion was confirmed by research results which indicated that MS patients had shown difficulties in evoking earlier presented stimuli, simultaneously having the ability to reconstruct facts from experimental material, under circumstances leading to recognition (Caine et al.: 1986; Carroll et al.: 1984; Rao et al.: 1986). The examined patients recalled less information from a text than people from random test groups (Caine et al.: 1986; Grant et al.: 1984; Rao et al.: 1984). They had worse results in reconstructing abstract syllables, words or word-pairs from a list, as well as in generating words belonging to a given semantic category (Grafman, Rao, Litvan: 1990; Mazurek, Szepietowska: 1992). MS patients had also difficulties with recalling nonverbal material, including geometric figures, chess patterns, points situated on fictitious maps. Yet these disorders were not as visible, as deficiencies in evoking verbal material.

In spite of the fact that results gathered from many studies acknowledge occurrence of difficulties in evoking material from the long-term memory among MS patients, lately researchers have also turned their attention towards observing these groups of people in assimilating new information. De Luca et al. (1994, 1998) had doubts about the hypothesis explaining the origin of memory deficiencies among MS patients only as a result of disturbance in recollection of memorized material. The authors have indicated that when controlling the number of memorized and reconstructed items there are no significant differences on the level of reconstructing previously memorized information between MS patients and randomly tested groups of healthy people, but for the fact, that patients need more stimuli exposures to be memorized in order to reach the level of training allowing for later reconstruction. This shows that MS patients have deficiencies on the level of acquiring information and not their evoking from the long-term memory. This regularity was visible both in the case of verbal (De Luca et al.: 1994, 1998) and nonverbal (De Luca et al.: 1998) material exposure, and at the same time, it is worth stressing that memory deficiencies in nonverbal tasks were not only connected with memorizing processes, but also concerned information storage.

A different approach to examining long-term memory disorders among MS patients is presented by Beatty et al. (1996). These authors divided groups of memory disorders among MS patients into three categories using method of statistical cluster analysis. The first group, amounting to 25% of all examined patients, consisted of people with no memory disorders. The second group (22%) were patients with serious memory impairments resembling amnesia. The last, biggest group (53%) had mild or moderate impairments. Thorton and Ratz (1997) emphasize the fact that the groups determined in the research by Beatty et al. (1996) may reflect stages of a deficiency continuum from mild to extremely serious disorders affecting MS patients.

Memory disorders among MS patients may be also treated as a result of disturbances in metamemory processing. The research outcomes presented by Beatty and Manson (1991) indicate that MS patients have difficulties in estimating their own memory capabilities along with impairments in planning and controlling cognitive processes. The authors assessed the abilities of MS patients for appropriate estimation of probability of their recollecting earlier presented information. The patients stated that their memory problems had not been confirmed in the actual tasks of evoking stimuli. The authors claim that this fact limits the possibility of using the method of subjective reports for estimating memory capabilities of MS patients.

Metamemory capabilities of MS patients were also analyzed in studies where an assessment of memory functions was done by the patients and their relatives. By juxtaposing the results Taylor et al. (1990) concluded that the appraisals of one's own memory capabilities provided by the patients are less adequate than the opinions presented by their relatives. Contradictory outcomes were submitted by Randolph, Arnett and Higginson (2001). Their research showed that evaluation of one's own memory problems, disclosed in subjective reports of MS patients, had been as accurate as the assessment done by their families, though the unanimity of the evaluations with the actual level of memory tasks had depended on the education of the respondents.

The connection between metacognitive processes and MS memory dysfunctions were proven also by research of Szepietowska (2002). In her studies MS patients used ineffective cognitive strategies, giving up semantic strategies to memorize a list of words, simultaneously carrying out only a superficial, phonetic analysis of the material. The author has put forward a hypothesis that ineffective memorization strategies may hinder the learning process, lengthen the time and increase the number of attempts needed to memorize a given text, as well as making it harder for a patient to bring out information from long-term memory. Inadequate strategies emerging already during the stage of coding may also encumber sending information to long-term memory (Szepietowska: 2002).

ATTENTION DISORDERS

Results of studies on attention disorders among MS patients do not allow explicitly to determine the intensification and range of these disorders and their relation to the course of the disease. Some of the research indicates that attention disorders may be the first symptom of cognitive deficiencies and, in some cases, they may occur in the earlier stages of MS (Lyon-Caen: 1986). Conversely, other authors did not observe any attention disorders among patients with neurological diseases in MS (Rao et al.: 1984). The studies dedicated to attention disorders among MS patients usually are based on the Symbol Digit Test. This test enables evaluating functioning of short-term memory and attention. The test is used in a version that requires a respondent to repeat a sequence of digits in a given order and in an adaptation when a respondent repeats the digits backwards. Beatty et al. (1995) using the task have proven that MS patients have a basic attention deficiency which distracts both ability to repeat the digits in a given order, as well as repeating them backwards. In their studies, Beatty et al. (1995) state that repeating digits backwards correlated more clearly with other cognitive impairments factors like category fluency, abstracting and memory tests. Beatty et al. (1995) suggest that such a correlation may be a result of an impact of one factor engaged in the carrying out of all the above-mentioned tasks. According to the authors the factor may be a damage in the divisibility of attention function.

Also Rao et al. (1991) used the task of repeating digits to evaluate the functioning of attention among MS patients. The examined patients had poorer results than people from a random test group only in the task of repeating digits backwards. No reduction in repeating the digits in a given order was observed. Similar results were achieved by D'Esposito et al. (1996). Deficiencies in attention among MS patients were also proven by research with the use of other types of tasks, including a verbal version of the Symbol Digit Modality Test (SDMT) and Paced Auditory Serial Addition Test (PASAT) (Litvan et al.: 1988).

THINKING AND MANAGEMENT FUNCTIONS DISORDERS

Thinking and executive functions disorders among MS patients include mainly problems regarding abstract thinking, deducting, planning and controlling complex cognitive activities, which is mirrored in the improper results of many neuropsychological tests, the Wisconsin Card Sorting Test (WCST) among others. The test checks the ability of a participant to display flexibility in abstract thinking by deducting the changing rules of the test and enables an evaluation of disorders in the area. In the WCST conducted by Heaton et. al (1985) MS patients made more perseveration errors than healthy people. This relation was characteristic for groups with chronic as well as secondary progressive course of the disease. Similar results were achieved by Rao et al. (1987). The authors confirmed a decline in abstract thinking among MS patients manifested by a lower number of achieved categories and a higher number of perseveration errors. The research by Rao et al. showed that the statistically significant differences concerned only people with chronic MS, whereas the results of the WCST among patients with decelerating-progressing course of MS were on a normal level. Lower results in creating categories during the WCST among MS patients and more explicit tendency to make perseveration errors in comparison to healthy people were also described by Beatty et al. (1995), Beatty and Manson (1996) and Arnett et al. (1994). The results achieved by Arnett et al. (1994) additionally emphasize the relation between difficulties in doing the WCST and damages in the frontal lobes area. This fact suggests that abstracting and problem-solving issues among MS patients may be caused by an inability to abandon a once learned strategy of responding, which ceases to be adequate. This conclusion is also supported by observations of MS patients who globally perform poorly in the WCST and yet have no problems in creating a first category (Beatty et al.: 1989; Rao et al.: 1987).

Beatty et al. have analyzed the potential influence of speech defects on the level of abstracting tasks. The authors compared the results achieved by MS patients in tasks needing verbal and nonverbal reasoning. MS patients performed poorer than healthy people both in verbal and nonverbal tasks which suggests that verbal disorders are not the only cause of difficulties in abstracting tasks. Beatty et. al (1994) have also juxtaposed results of MS patients with healthy people on a similar level of linguistic competence and proved that MS patients, in spite of their preserved verbal skills, had performed poorer in abstracting tasks than healthy people. MS patients achieved worse results in other tests evaluating conceptual and abstract thinking together with switching between mental categories, such as the California Card Sorting Test (Beatty et al.: 1995; Beatty and Manson: 1996), the Levine Concept Formation Task (Rao, Hammeke: 1984) or the Category Test (Heaton et al.: 1985).

Another group of studies dedicated to executive functions among MS patients are tests on memorizing the order of arranged stimuli. The fact of MS patients having difficulties evoking earlier presented lists of words was confirmed by Armstrong (1996) along with Beatty and Manson (1991). Different results of executive functions studies among MS patients were presented by Arnett et al. (1997). The subjects did not differ from healthy people in terms of tasks requiring memorizing lists of words put into semantic subgroups of various numbers. In the same research Arnett et al. (1997) claim that MS patients have problems with effective usage of information on semantic categories and planning abilities, measured by the Tower of Hanoi puzzle.

Speech Impairments

Speech impairments among MS patients boil down mainly to dysarthria. Its incidence among MS patients amounts to 40-50% (Hartelius et al.: 2000, Sandyk: 1995). The most common symptoms of dysarthria among MS patients are dyspnea, problems with vocal emission, prosodic disorders of speech rhythm, accent and volume, scanning speech and monotony. The type and intensity of dysarthria symptoms are varied and seem to depend on the course of the disease and its duration (Hartelius et al.: 2000). MS patients also display problems in relation to identifying their own emotions expressed by prosodic features of speech, not resulting from aphasia, depression or hearing impairments (Beatty, Orbelo, Sorocco, Ros: 2003).

In few cases of MS patients aphasia caused by extent demyelination lesions situated in the dominant hemisphere was observed (Vilaverde-Gonzalesi et al.: 2003). Its incidence amounts to 0.7-3% of MS patients (Achiron et al.: 1992; Lacour, De Seze: 2004). Aphasia is usually accompanied by a new attack of the disease and is short-lived and temporary in nature. Most frequently it is a motor aphasia, rarely its sensory or amnesic type (Rao,

Callanan: 1991, Di Majo et al.: 2001; Vilaverde-Gonzalesi et al.: 2003). Also such phenomena as auditory agnosia, oral apraxia, dysgraphia or dyslexia hardly ever occur (Merson, Rolnick: 1998; Szepietowska: 1997). These dysfunctions are usually diagnosed in people with Schilder's disease – a specific type of MS. In very few cases of MS alexia (Dagulu et al.: 1996; Shiota et al.: 1989) and agraphia (Day et al.: 1987; Mao-Draayer, Panitch: 2004) are also present.

Speed of Information Processing

A characteristic feature of cognitive functioning among MS patients is the presence of bradyphrenia and bradykinesia, manifested in all psychological tasks regardless of their modality. On the basis of conducted research it is still hard to say whetherslowness of information processing is caused by motor retardation or the other way around.

Deterioration or discontinuity of nerve conduction due to demyelination hampers motor tasks and leads to lengthening of motor activities included in cognitive functions tests. The slowness may also be an outcome of structural and functional discontinuity of cortical and subcortical junctions in the brain, resulting in cognitive impairments of a patient, hindering stimuli identification, information transfer within the nervous system, reply choice, performance control. Also studies with use of evoked potentials showed a correlation between pathological changes in the area of P300 potential and deterioration in cognitive capabilities manifested in the psychological tests. In the research of Newton et al. (1989) slowness or absence of P300 component among MS patients was connected with decline in results of psychological tests measuring intellectual performance, verbal and nonverbal memory. Similar outcomes were achieved by Honing, Ramsay, Sheremata (1992). It is worth stressing that besides the negative influence on neuropsychological tests, slowness of information processing and motor retardation hinder functioning of MS patients in everyday situations which results in decline of their work efficiency as well as quality of life (Bagert, Camplair, Bourdette: 2002).

Clinical Variables and MS Cognitive Impairments

Clinical data indicate that MS cognitive impairments are dependent on the influence of clinical variables, such as course of disease, its duration, the intensity of neurological disorders and accompanied dysphoria.

Course of MS and Cognitive Impairments

The spread character of the demyelination lesions causes the course and clinical picture of MS to be highly differentiated. The disease may have a relapsing-remitting course which is characterized by sudden new attacks of the disease and remissions of symptoms or a secondary progressive course which leads to early new attacks of the disease, resulting in a chronic progressive course – originally progressing without remissions or sudden new attacks of the disease (Szepietowska: 1997).

Nocentini et al. (2006) have proven a frequent occurrence of cognitive disorders of various intensity in terms of pace and memory among patients with a relapsing-remitting course of MS. Similar results were achieved by Heaton et al. (1985), Van der Burg et al. (1987) and Zivadinov et al. (2001). Yet most of the clinic data point to a global decline in cognitive capabilities being a characteristic feature especially among patients with chronic or secondary progressive MS (Beatty et al.: 1988; 1989, Heaton et al.: 1985; Feinstein et al.: 1992). The results achieved by patients in standardized neuropsychological test indicate that cognitive disorders occur among 50% patients with a relapsing-remitting MS while the rate among chronic MS patients is over 90% (Heaton et al.: 1985; Rao et al.: 1984; Sandyk: 1997). It means that patients with advanced neurological symptoms typically are under negative, non-remissive cognitive impairments.

Monitoring the chronic group of MS patients reveals also differences in the intensity of cognitive deficiencies from mild and selective disturbances in notional memory through moderate memory impairments up to serious dementia syndromes (Rao et al.: 1987). Comi et al. (1995) have proven that impairments of memory, attention, speech, executive functions and visual functions occur more often among patients with a secondary progressing MS in comparison to people who have primary progressing MS. Wachowius et al. (2005) gathered results showing a poorer level of answers to tests for verbal learning and fluency among progressive MS than the level of secondary progressive MS patients. Whereas Foong et al. (2000) did not disclose significant differences concerning memory and cognitive functioning between patients having chronic and secondary progressive MS, although these both groups achieved poorer results in cognitive tasks than healthy people from a random control group.

The diversity of results regarding the relation between the course of disease and types as well as intensity of MS-related cognitive impairments reflects methodological problems of research in this field. An analysis of MS influence on cognitive symptoms among patients is hindered by some early results of MS researchers who employed other criteria of measuring course of disease or omitting this factor on the level of patients' selection for testing. As a consequence they analyzed altogether results of people with different course of MS, who achieved diverse, sometimes even contradictory results in neuropsychological tests. Another factor adding to the lack of cohesion in the results was using different methods of cognitive impairment evaluation (Nocentini et al.: 2006).

Studies concerning a relation between duration of disease and intensity of cognitive impairments also do not lead to finite conclusions. In some cases cognitive impairments occur in the earlier stages of the disease and precede neurological disorders (Lyon-Caen et al.: 1986), other cases show no cognitive impairments even when in the course of the disease patients become physically disabled (Pozzili et al.: 1993).

Most of patients in the early stage of the disease achieves poorer results than healthy people in abstract thinking and problem-solving tests (Ruggieri et al.: 2003). Patients with early stages of MS also suffered from dementia syndromes, but such serious disorders are extremely rare and the lesions underlying are yet to be thoroughly analyzed and described (Amato, Zipoli: 2003).

The majority of long-term research conducted in order to evaluate the development of cognitive deficiencies in the course of disease have proven a gradual increase of memory, attention and learning disorders correlating with progressing demyelination lesions, health deterioration, age of patients and chronic course of MS. Amato and Zipoli (2003) stated that the prevalence rate of cognitive impairments among examined people has risen from 26% to 56% during a period of 10 years from the first research. Similar results were achieved by Zivadinov et al. (2001) who juxtaposed the data in 2-year intervals. The actual relationship between the duration of the disease and intensification of cognitive impairments was not confirmed by all studies. A neuropsychological test analysis of 44 MS patients done by Hohola et al. (1997) revealed that only 4 out of all subjects had poorer results than a year ago, 19 performed better, while the cognitive level of 21 patients was not subject to change. Also Lynch, Parmenter and Denney (2005) did not find any proof confirming a connection between the duration of the disease and deterioration of cognitive functioning among MS patients.

The Extent of Intensification in Neurological Dysfunctions and MS Cognitive Impairments

Research on influence of neurological state of MS patients on their cognitive impairments also do not allow to formulate any clear-cut conclusions. One may quote some studies that show high results on Kurtzke's DS and EDS Scales as an indicative of the extent of intensification in neurological disorders. These results also correlate with verbal and nonverbal memory impairments and declined abstracting capability (Grant et al.: 1984; Heaton et al.: 1985; Minden et al.: 1990). Thorton and Ratz (1997) basing their research on meta-analysis of MS memory disorders confirmed that patients with higher scores in EDSS and DSS achieve poorer results in free evoking tests in comparison to a group of patients with lower scalar results. A strong correlation between an intensification of cognitive deficiencies and the extent of physical disability was also discovered by Lynch, Parmenter and Denney (2005). This dependence was characteristic for both people in the early stage of the disease as well as patients having MS with duration of 10 or more years. This significant correlation between EDSS results and outcomes of neuropsychological tests enabled the authors to come to a conclusion that there is a possibility to predict the extent of damage for cognitive processes on the basis of data regarding physical disability. However, these data were not confirmed by research carried out by other authors. Rao et al. (1991) have observed only a slight dependence between a neurological state and cognitive impairments, whereas Marsh (1980) claimed there is a correlation between the duration of the disease and results of Kurtzke's Scales but no such dependence exists between verbal functions or global intellectual capability measured by the Wechsler Scale of Intelligence and results of EDSS.

Szepietowska (1997) underlines the fact that establishing a relationship between the extent of neurological disorders and the degree of cognitive dysfunctions by means of DS and EDS Scales may be doubtful. The scales concentrate on evaluation of motor activities and a small percentage of them enables to assess activities of these structures in the nervous system which mediate in the course of cognitive processes. More useful tools for monitoring disabilities and disorders among MS patients are these including not only physical but also psychological and social functioning of a patient, including scales measuring quality of life of patients (FAMS, SF – 36, MSQOL – 540) (Vickrey et al.: 1995; Ware, Sherbourne: 1992).

There exists also a group of studies aiming at the relation of the image and intensity of cognitive impairments among MS patients to the extent and localization of demyelination lesions in the nervous system (Arnett et al.: 1994; Rao et al.: 1991). The results of this research indicate that the area damaged by demyelination is more extensive in a group of patients with no memory, abstract thinking disorders, verbal fluency or spatial awareness disorders (Rao et al.: 1991; Fischer et al.: 2000). The heaviest cognitive impairments and intense dementia syndromes accompany damages in the area of commissura magna (Rao et al.: 1991; Swirsky-Sacchetti et al.: 1992). MS patients with such lesions have serious cognitive impairments (Szepietowska, 1997) and the occurrence of atrophy in commissura magna enables patients to be differentiated into patients with dementia and patients with mild cognitive impairments. Research by Arnett et al. (1994) have shown a significant correlation between abstract thinking disorders and the extent of damage in the frontal lobe area. Patients with demyelination lesions in the frontal lobe area had more difficulties in solving tasks from the Wisconsin Card Sorting Test and made more mistakes, including perseveration errors, in comparison to people with disseminated lesions and people with small surface of lesions. MS patients have shown problems with planning their own cognitive actions and their control, as well as knowledge on the relationship between memory effects and inner and outer factors (Beatty, Manson: 1991; Mazurek, Szepietowska: 1992). Also Foong (1997) have confirmed the connection between the performance in cognitive tests and intensification of demyelination lesions in the frontal lobe area. The data was also confirmed by neuroimaging research which proved the relation of MS with hypermetabolism in the frontal lobe area (Brooks: 1991). Since frontal lobe abnormalities are not a symptom specific to MS and is present during other diseases of the nervous system, hypermetabolism of these organs has an indirect role rather than being the prime mover of clinical overview of cognitive impairments.

According to other authors the abnormalities of cognitive processes are most of all connected with damage of subcortical structures (Cendrowski: 1993; Rao: 1991). A clinical profile of MS cognitive impairments suits the symptoms of the subcortical dementia resulting from damages to the axial areas of the brain stem, thalamus or medulla as disorders in subcortical structure are relatively often occur among MS patients.

Studies done in the recent years show that MS demyelination is not a focal process and subtle changes in both the myelin sheath and axial fiber, include also the normal-appearing brain tissue (NABT) (Filippi et al.: 2000). These lesions arise in the most earliest stages of the disease and it is supposed that they may precede structural changes (Rovaris et al.: 2000). Preliminary studies suggest that early cognitive impairments may result from the subtle changes in NABT rather than from focal changes (Rovaris et al.: 1998; Benedict, Carone, Bakshi: 2004). A correlative analysis done by Zivadinov (2001) acknowledged a strong association between cognitive impairments tests and brain atrophy with intensification of NABT microlesions. Nowadays scientists frequently stress the fact that MS pathological lesions may also afflict the gray matter including the neocortex (Dalton et al.: 2004). Amato has observed a significant correlation between the extent of atrophy in the cerebral cortex and test results concerning attention, verbal memory and fluency. At the same time it is worth stressing that the atrophy was diagnosed only among patients with cognitive impairments (Amato: 2004).

The Influence of Depression on Cognitive Functioning Among MS Patients

It seems that MS cognitive impairments may be additionally strengthened by emotional disorders of patients. Especially MS-characteristic memory problems may deepen under the influence of dysphoria, very common among patients. The coexistence of mood changes with cognitive impairments may also effect the perception of patient's own cognitive abilities.

Even some early psychological research on MS has proven that MS patients achieve higher results in tests measuring their level of anxiety and depression in comparison to people of similar or heavier physical disability (Whitlock, Siskind: 1980). Emotional disorders among MS patients seems to have a complex etiology. Some of the mood changes are symptoms of adjustment disturbances – a response of the organism to a difficult psychological situation of a patient suffering from a chronic disease restricting motor fitness. Neuroanatomical data indicate damages in the brain tissue as the cause of major depression among MS patients (Sabatini et al.: 1996). Lifetime prevalence of depression among MS patients is greater than in all of the population or people suffering from other neurological diseases (Schubert, Foliart: 1993; Kessler et al.: 1994) and amounts to around 50% (Feinstein, Feinstein: 2001, Minden, Schiffer: 1990). The symptoms of depression are seen even in patients with a very mild type of MS (Sullivan et al.: 1995a, 1995b).

The problem of dependence between depression and cognitive impairment among MS patients was undertaken in a few studies. Gilchrist and Creed (1994) have stated that dysphoria among MS patients is connected with impairments of cognitive activities. The examined patients diagnosed as having MS and depression achieved poorer results in verbal learning and intellectual functioning tests than patients without depression. The authors claim that depression among patients increases, when cognitive impairments become the reason of professional difficulties or interpersonal problems.

Arnett et al. (1999) have demonstrated a negative influence of depression on tests regarding attention capacity done by MS patients, while Thorton and Ratz (1997) in their meta-analysis of memory research during MS proved correct the connection between the results achieved by patients in the Beck Depression Inventory and the outcomes of working memory tests. Yet these studies do not give a consistent answer whether dysphoria strengthens cognitive deficiencies or do patients realizing their memory and attention disorders fall into depression. The issue has to be studied further, especially that there are many reports showing no obvious connection between depression and cognitive impairments in MS (Moller et al.: 1994; Grafman et al.: 1991; Good et al.: 1992, Rao, Leo, St. Aubin-Faubert: 1989) or the results were of no statistical value (Rao, Leo, Bernardin, Unverzagt: 1991).

Bruce and Arnett (2004) have studied the influence of depression on subjective evaluation of own cognitive capabilities among MS patients. The authors have analyzed relations concerning the extent of memory disorders gathered from MS patients who were diagnosed for mild, moderate or serious depression and those who had no dysphoria. People suffering from mild depression showed a tendency to underestimate their own memory abilities in objective neuropsychological tests, while people with no depression overestimated them. Whereas patients with moderate depression have evaluated their memory abilities correspondingly to the results of objective memory measurements. The authors interpreted the results in the context of Beck's cognitive theory of depression and the depressive realism hypothesis.

Psychological literature begins to give a lot of space to cognitive impairments among patients suffering from MS. It is accepted that this type of abnormality may be of great importance to the clinical overview of the disease and to quality of life of patients.

The results of research done so far did not give clear-cut answers regarding the incidence, clinical view, intensity and course of cognitive deficiencies in MS. There is also little information about the pathomechanism behind these impairments and their influence on the rehabilitation of patients.

References

Achiron, A., Ziv, I., Djaldetti, R., Goldberg, H., Krutzky, A. & Melamed, E. (1992). Aphasia in multiple sclerosis: Clinical and radiologic correlations. *Neurology, 42*, 2195 – 2197.

Amato, M.P. & Zipoli, V. (2003). Clinical management of cognitive impairment in multiple sclerosis: A review of current evidence. *International MS Journal,* 10, 72 – 83.

Amato, M.P., Bartolozzi, M.L., Zipoli, V. Portaccio, E., Mortilla, M., Guidi, L., Siracusa, G, Sorbi, S., Federico, A. & De Stefano, N. (2004). Neurocortical volume decrease in relapsing – remitting MS patients with mild cognitive impairment, *Neurology, 13*, 89 – 93.

Armstrong, C., Onishi, K., Robinson, K., D'Esposito, M., Thompson, H., Rostami, A. & Grossman, M. (1996). Serial position and temporal cue effects in multiple sclerosis: Two subtypes of defective memory mechanisms. *Neuropsychologia, 34,* 853 – 862.

Arnett, P., Rao, S., Bernardin, L. Grafman, J., Yetkin, F. Lobeck, L. (1994). Relationship between frontal lobe lesions and Wisconsin Card Sorting Test performance in patients with multiple sclerosis. *Neurology, 44*, 420 – 425.

Arnett, P.A., Grafman, J., Rao, S.M., Bernardin, L. & Luchetta, T. (1997). Executive functions in multiple sclerosis: An analysis of temporal ordering, semantic encoding, and planning abilities. *Neuropsychology, 11*, 535 – 544.

Arnett, P.A., Higginson, C.I., Voss, W.D., Wright, B., Bender, W.I., Wurst, J.M. & Tippin, J.M. (1999). Depressed mood in multiple sclerosis: Relationship to capacity – demanding memory and attentional functioning. *Neuropsychology, 13,* 434 – 446.

Bagert, B., Camplair, P. & Bourdette, D. (2002). Cognitive dysfunction in multiple sclerosis. *Therapy in Practice, 16,* 445 – 455.

Beatty, P.A. & Gange, J.J. (1977). Neuropsychological aspects of multiple sclerosis. *Journal of Nervous and Mental Disease, 164*, 42 – 50.

Beatty, W.W. & Monson, N. (1991). Metamemory in multiple sclerosis. *Journal of Clinical and Experimental Neuropsychology, 13,* 309 – 327.

Beatty, W.W. & Monson, N. (1996). Picture and motoring sequencing in multiple sclerosis. *Journal of Clinical and Experimental Neuropsychology, 16,* 165 – 172.

Beatty, W.W., Goodkin, D.E., Beatty, P.A. & Monson, N. (1989). Frontal lobe dysfunction and memory impairment in patients with chronic progressive multiple sclerosis. *Brain and Cognition, 11*, 73 – 86.

Beatty, W.W., Goodkin, D.E., Monson, N. & Beatty, P.A. (1989). Cognitive disturbances in patients with relapsing – remitting multiple sclerosis. *Archives of Neurology, 46*, 1113 – 1119.

Beatty, W.W., Goodkin, D.E., Monson, N., Beatty, P.A. & Hertsgaard, D. (1988). Anterograde and retrograde amnesia in patients with chronic progressive multiple sclerosis. *Archives of Neurology, 45*, 611 – 619.

Beatty, W.W., Hames, K.A., Blanco, C.R., Paul, R.H. & Wilbanks, S.L. (1995). Verbal abstraction deficits in multiple sclerosis. Neuropsychology. 9, 198 – 205.

Beatty, W.W., Orbelo, D.M., Sorocco, K.H. & Ross, E.D. (2003). Comprehension of affective prosody in multiple sclerosis. *Multiple Sclerosis, 9,* 148 – 153.

Beatty, W.W., Paul, R.H., Blanco, C.R., Hames, K.A., S.L. (1995). Attention in multiple sclerosis: correlates of impairment on WAIS – R Digit Span Test. *Applied Neuropsychology, 2,* 139 – 144.

Beatty, W.W., Wilbanks, S.L. Blanco, C.R., Hames, K.A., Tivis, R. & Paul, R.H. (1996). Memory disturbance in multiple sclerosis: Reconsideration of patterns of performance on the Selective Reminding Test. *Journal of Clinical and Experimental Neuropsycholog, 18,* 56 – 62.

Benedict, R.H., Carone, D.A. & Bakshi, R. (2004). Correlation brain atrophy with cognitive dysfunction, mood disturbances, and personality disorder in multiple sclerosis. *Journal of Neuroimaging, 14 (3 Suppl),* 36 – 45.

Brassington, J.C. & Marsh, N.V. (1998). Neuropsychological aspects of multiple sclerosis. *Neuropsychology Review, 8*, 43 – 77.

Brooks, D. (1991). PET – its clinical role in neurology. *Journal of Neurology, Neurosurgery, and Psychiatry, 54,* 1 – 5.

Bruce, J.M., Arnett, P.A. (2004). Self – reported everyday memory and depression in patients with multiple sclerosis. *Journal of Clinical and Experimental Neuropsychology,* 26, 200 – 214.

Caine, E.D., Bamford, K.A., Schiffer, R.B., Shoulson, L. & Levy, S. (1986). A controlled neuropsychological comparison of Huntington's disease and multiple sclerosis. *Archives of Neurology, 43*, 249 – 254.

Carroll, M., Gates, R. & Roldan, F. (1984). Memory impairment in multiple sclerosis. *Neuropsychologia, 22,* 297 – 302.

Cendrowski, W. (1993). *Stwardnienie rozsiane*. Warszawa, PZWL.

Comi, G., Filippi, M., Martinelli, V., Campi, A., Rodegher, M., Alberoni, M., Sirabian, G. & Canal, N. (1995). Brain MRI correlates of cognitive impairment in primary and secondary progressive multiple sclerosis. *Journal of The Neurological Science, 132*, 222 – 227.

D'Esposito, M., Onishi, K., Thompson, H., Robinson, K. Armstrong, C., Grossman, M. (1996). Working memory impairments in multiple sclerosis: Evidence from dual – task paradigm. *Neuropsychology, 10,* 51 – 56.

Dalton, C.M., Chard, D.T., Davies, G.R., Miszkiel, K.A., Altmann, D.R., Fernando, K., Plant, G.T., Thompson, A.J. & Miller, D.H. (2004). Early development of multiple sclerosis in associated with progressive grey matter atrophy in patients presenting with clinically isolated syndromes. *Brain, 127,* 1101 – 1107.

Day, T.J., Fisher, A.G. & Mastaglia, F.L. (1987). Alexia with agraphia in multiple sclerosis. *Journal of the Neurological Sciences, 78*, 343 – 348.

DeLuca, J. , Batrbieri – Berger, S. & Johnson, S.K. (1994).The nature of memory impairment in multiple sclerosis: acquisition versus retrieval. *Journal of Clinical and Experimental Neuropsychology, 16,* 183 – 185.

DeLuca, J., Gaudino, E.A., Diamond, B.J., Christodoulou, C. & Engel, R.A. (1988). Acquisition and storage deficits in multiple sclerosis. *Journal of Clinical and Experimental Neuropsychology, 3*, 376 – 390.

Di Majo, L., Bisceglia, M., Lanzillo, R., D'Angelo, V., Gorgoglione, L., Chiacchio, L. & Orefice, G. (2002). Aphasia as a rare presentation of monosymptomatic demyelinating disease: case report and review of literature. *Neurological sciences: official journal of the Italian Neurological Society and of the Italian Society of Clinical Neurophysiology, 23,* 79 – 82.

Dogulu, C.F., Lamsi, T. & Karabudak, R., Alexia without agraphia in multiple sclerosis. *Journal of Neurology, Neurosurgery, and Psychiatry, 61,* 528.

Feinstein, A. & Feinstein, K. (2001). Depression associated with multiple sclerosis: Looking beyond diagnosis to symptom expression, *Journal of Affective Disorders, 66,* 193 – 198.

Feinstein, A. (1995). Cognitive dysfunction in multiple sclerosis. *International MS Journal, 1995, 2*, 61 – 67.

Feinstein, A. (2004). The neuropsychiatry of multiple sclerosis. Canadian journal of Psychiatry, 49, 157 – 163.

Feinstein, A. (2006). Mood disorders in multiple sclerosis and the effects on cognition. *Journal of The Neurological Sciences, 245*, 63 – 66

Feinstein, A., Kartsounis, L.D., miller, D.H., Youl, B.D. & Ron, M.A. (1992). Clinically isolated lesions of the type seen in multiple sclerosis: A cognitive, psychiatric, and MRI follow up study. *Journal of Neurology, Neurosurgery, and Psychiatry, 55*, 869 – 876.

Filippi, M., Tortorella, C., Rovaris, M., Bozzali, M., Possa, F., Sormani, M.P., Iannucci, G. Comi, G. (2000). Changes in the normal appearing brain tissue and cognitive impairment in multiple sclerosis. *Journal of Neurology, Neurosurgery, and Psychiatry. 68*, 157 – 161.

Fischer, J.S. (1988). Using the Wechsler Memory Scale – Revised to detect and characterize memory deficits in multiple sclerosis. *The Clinical Neuropsychologist, 2,* 149 – 172.

Fischer, J.S., Priore, R.L., Jacobs, L.D., Cookfair, D.L., Rudick, R.A., Herndon, R.M., Richert, J.R., Salazar, A.M., Goodkin, D.E., Granger, C.V., Simon, J.H., Grafman, J.H., Lezak, M.D., O'Reilly Hovey, K.M., Perkins, K.K., Barilla-Clark, D., Shacter, M., Shucard, D.W., Davidson, A.L., Wende, K.E., Bourdette, D.N. & Kooijmans-Coutinho, M.F. (2000). Neuropsychological effects of interferon beta-1a in relapsing multiple sclerosis. Multiple Sclerosis Collaborative Research Group. *Annals of Neurology, 48*, 885 – 92.

Foong, J., Rozewicz, I., Quaghebeur, G., Dave, C.A., Kartsounis, L.D., Thompson, A.J., Miller, D.H. & Ron, M.A. (1997). Executive function in multiple sclerosis. The role of frontal lobe pathology. *Brain, 120,* 15 – 26.

Foong, J., Rozewicz, L., Chong, W.K., Thompson, A.J., Miller, D.H. & Ron, M.A. (2000). A comparison of neuropsychological deficits in primary and secondary progressive multiple sclerosis. *Journal of Neurology, 274,* 97 – 101.

Gilchrist, A.C. & Creed, F.H. (1994). Depression, cognitive impairment and social stress in multiple sclerosis. *Journal of Psychosomatic Research, 38,* 193 – 201.

Grafman, J., Rao, S.M. & Litvan, I. (1990). Disorders of memory. In S.M. Rao (Ed.), *Neurobehavioral aspects of multiple sclerosis* (pp. 102 – 117). New York: Oxford University Press.

Grafman, J., Rao, S.M., Bernardin, L. & Leo, G.J. (1991). Automatic memory processes in patients with multiple sclerosis. *Archives of Neurology, 48,* 1072 – 1075.

Grant, I., McDonald, W.I., Trimble, M.R., Smith, E. & Reed, R. (1984). Deficient learning and memory in early and middle phases of multiple sclerosis. *Journal of Neurology, Neurosurgery, and Psychiatry, 47,* 250 – 255.

Hartelius, L., Runmarker, B., Andersen, O. & Nord, L. (200). Temporal speech characteristic of individuals with multiple sclerosis and ataxic dysarthria: 'scanning speech' revisited. *Folia Phoniatrica Et logopaedia: Official Organ Of The International Association Of Logopedics And Phoniatric (IALP), 52*, 228 – 238. Abstract.

Heaton, R.K., Nelson, L.M., Thompson, D.S., Burks, J.S. & Franklin, G.M. (1985). Neuropsychological findings in relapsing – remitting and chronic – progressive multiple sclerosis. *Journal of Consulting and Clinical Psychology, 53*, 103 – 110.

Hohol, M.J., Guttman, C.R. & Orav, J. (1997). Serial neuropsychological assessment and magnetic resonance imaging analysis in multiple sclerosis. *Archives of Neurology, 54,* 1018 – 1025.

Honing, L.S., Rasmsay, R.E. & Sheremata, W.A. (1992). Event – related potential P300 in multiple sclerosis. Relation to magnetic resonance imaging and cognitive impairment. *Archives of Neurology, 49,* 44 – 50.

Kessler, R.C., McGonagle, K.A., Zhao, S. & Nelson, C.B. (1994). Lifetime and 12 month prevalence of DSM-III- R psychiatric disorders in United States. Results from the National Co – Morbidity Survey. *Archives of General Psychiatry, 51*, 8 – 19.

Lacour, A., de Seze, J., Revenco, E., Lebrun, C., Masmoudi, K., Vidry, E., Rumbach, L., Chatel, M., Verier, A. & Vermersch, P. (2004). Acute aphasia in multiple sclerosis: a multicenter study of 22 patients. *Neurology, 62*, 974 – 977.

Litvan, I., Grafman, J., Vendrell, P., Martinez, J.M., Junque, C., Vendrell, J.M. & Barraquer – Bordas, J.L. 91988). Multiple memory deficits in patients with multiple sclerosis: Exploring the working memory system. Archives of Neurology, 45, 607 – 610.

Lynch, S.G., Parmenter, B.A. & Douglas, R.D. (2005). The association between cognitive impairment and physical disability in multiple sclerosis. *Multiple Sclerosis, 11,* 469 – 476.

Lyon – Caen, O., Jouvet, R. & Hauser, S. (1986). Cognitive function in recent onset demyelinating diseases. *Neurology, 40,* 900 – 903.

Mao – Draayer, Y. & Panitch, H. (2004). Alexia without agraphia in multiple sclerosis: case report with magnetic resonance imaging localization, *Multiple Sclerosis, 10*, 705 – 707.

Marsh, G. (1980). Disability and intellectual function in multiple sclerosis. Journal of Nervous and Mental Disease, 168, 758 – 762.

Marsh, G. (1980). Disability and intellectual function in multiple sclerosis patients. The *Journal of Nervous and Mental Disease, 168,* 758 – 762.

Mazurek, B., Szepietowska, E.M. (1992). Problemy mnestyczne chorych na MS – psychologiczne badania eksperymentalne. *Annales,* Sekcja J, UMCS, Wydz. Ped. i Psych., V, 8, 103 – 116.

Merson, R.M. & Rolnick, M.I. (1998). Speech – language pathology and dysphagia in multiple sclerosis. Physical Medicine And Rehabilitation Clinics of North America, 9, 631 – 641. Abstract.

Minden, S.L. & Schiffer, R.B. (1990). Affective disorders in multiple sclerosis: Review and recommendations for clinical research. *Archives of Neurology, 47,* 98 – 104.

Minden, S.L., Moes, E.J., Orav, J., Kaplan, E. & reich, P. (1990). Memory impairment in multiple sclerosis. *Journal of Clinical and Experimental Neuropsychology, 12*, 566 – 586.

Newton, M.R., Barret, G., Callanan, M.M. & Towell, A.D. Cognitive event- related potentials in multiple sclerosis, *Brain, 112* (Pt 6), 1637 – 1660.

Nocentini, U., Pasqualetti, P., Bonavita, S., Buccafusca, M., De Caro, M.F., Farina, D., Girlanda, P., Le Pira, F., Lugaresi, A., Quattrone, A., Reggio, A., Salemi, G., Savettieri, G., Tedeschi, G., Trojano, M., Valentino, P. & Caltagirone, C. (2006). Cognitive dysfunction in patients with relapsing – remitting multiple sclerosis. *Multiple Sclerosis, 12,* 77 – 87.

Parmenter, B.A., Denney, D.R. & Lynch, S.G. (2003). The cognitive performance of patients with multiple sclerosis during periods of high and low fatigue, *Multiple Sclerosis, 9*, 111 – 118.

Pozzilli, C., Passafiume, D. & Bemardi, S. (1993). Anatomical and functional correlate of cognitive deficit in multiple sclerosis. *Journal of The Neurological Sciences, 1993*, 115 (Suppl.), 55 – 58.

Randolph, J.J., Arnett, P.A. & Higginson, C.J. (2001). Metamemory and tested cognitive functioning in multiple sclerosis. *The Clinical Neuropsychologist, 15*, 357 – 368.

Rao, S., Grafman, J., DiGiulio, D., Mittenberg, W., Bernardin, L., Leo, G., Luchetta, T. & Unverzagt F. (1993). Memory dysfunction in multiple sclerosis: Its relation to working memory, semantic encoding, and implicit learning. *Neuropsychology, 7,* 364 – 374.

Rao, S.M. (1986). Neuropsychology of multiple sclerosis: A critical review. *Journal of Clinical and Experimental Neuropsychology, 8,* 503 – 542.

Rao, S.M., Hammeke, T.A. & Speech, T.J. (1987). Wisconsin Card Sorting Test performance in relapsing – remitting and chronic – progressive multiple sclerosis. *Journal of Consulting and Clinical Psychology, 55*, 263 – 265.

Rao, S.M., Hammeke, T.A., McQuillen, M.P., Khatri, B.O. & Lloyd, D. (1984). Memory disturbance in chronic progressive multiple sclerosis. *Archives of Neurology, 41*, 625 – 631.

Rao, S.M., Leo, G.J., Bernardin, L. & Unverzagt, F. (1991). Cognitive dysfunction in multiple sclerosis: I. Frequency, patterns, and prediction, *Neurology, 41,* 685 – 691.

Ron, M.A. & Callanan, M. (1991). Cognitive abnormalities in MS: a psychometric and MRI study. *Psychological Medicine, 21,* 59 – 68.

Rovaris, M. & Filippi, M. (2000). MRI correlates of cognitive dysfunction in multiple sclerosis patients. *Journal of Neurovirology, 6,* 172 – 175.

Rovaris, M. & Filippi, M., Falautano, M. Minicucci, L., Rocca, M.A., Martinelli, V. & Comi, G. (1998). Relation between MR abnormalities and patterns of cognitive impairment in multiple sclerosis, *Neurology, 50,* 1601 – 1608.

Ruggieri, R.M., Palermo, R., Gennuso, M., Settipani, N. & Piccoli, F. (2003). Cognitive impairments in patient suffering from relapsing – remitting multiple sclerosis with EDSS<or=3.5. *Acta Neurologica Scandinavica. 108,* 323- 326.

Sabatini, L., Pozzilli, C., Pantano, P., Koudriavtseva, T. (1996). Involvement of the limbic system in multiple sclerosis patients with depressive disorders. *Biological Psychiatry, 39,* 970 – 975.

Sandyk, R. (1995). Reversal of alexia in multiple sclerosis by weak electromagnetic fields. *International Journal of Neurocience, 83*, 69 – 79.

Schubert, R.S.B. & Foliart, R.H. (1993). Increased depression in multiple sclerosis a meta – analys. *Psychosomatics, 34,* 124 – 130.

Shiota, J., Sugita, K. Kikushima, S., Maki, T. & Takeuchi, T. (1989). A case of multiple sclerosis with pure alexia. *No To Shinkei. Brain And Nerve, 41*, 961 – 964. Abstract.

Sullivan, M.J., Weinshenker, B., Mikail, S., Bishop, S.R. (1995a). Screening for major depression in the early stages of multiple sclerosis. *The Canadian Journal of Neurological Sciences, 22,* 228 – 231.

Sullivan. M.J., Weinshenker, B., Mikail, S., Edgley, K. (1995b). Depression before and after diagnosis of multiple sclerosis. *Multiple Sclerosis, 1,* 104 – 108.

Swirsky – Sacchetti, T., Mitchell, D., Seward, J. Gonzales, C., Lublin, F., Knobler, R. & Field, H.L. (1992). Neuropsychological and structural brain lesions in multiple sclerosis: A regional analysis. *Neurology, 42,* 1291 – 1295.

Szepietowska, E..M. (2002). Deficyt strategii pamięciowych u osób chorych na stwardnienie rozsiane (SM). *Przegląd Psychologiczny, 45,* 347 – 359.

Szepietowska, E.M. (1997). Zaburzenia w funkcjonowaniu poznawczym chorych na stwardnienie rozsiane. In A. Herzyk, & D. Kądzielawa (Eds), *Związek mózg – zachowanie w ujęciu neuropsychologii klinicznej* (217 – 246). Lublin. UMCS

Taylor, R. (1990). Relationships between cognitive test performance and everyday cognitive difficulties in multiple sclerosis. *British Journal of Clinical Psychology, 29*, 251 – 252.

Thorton, A.E. & Raz, N. (1997). Memory impairment in multiple sclerosis: A quantitative review. *Neuropsychology, 11*, 357 – 366.

Van der Burg, W., van Zomeren, A.H., Minderhoud, J.M., Prange, A.J. & Meijer, N.S.A. (1987). Cognitive impairment in patients with multiple sclerosis and mild physical disability. *Archives of Neurology, 44,* 494 – 501.

Vickrey, B.G., Hays, R.D., Harooni, R. & Myers, L.W. (1995). A health - related quality of life measure for multiple sclerosis. *Quality of Life Research: An International Journal of Quality of Life Aspects of Treatment, Care & Rehabilitation, 4,* 187 – 206.

Vilaverde –González, R., Fernández – Villalba, E., Moreno – Escribano, A., Alias – Linares, E. & Garcia – Santos, J.M. (2003). Foreign language syndrome as a first sign of multiple sclerosis. *Revista De Neurologia, 36,* 1035 – 1039. Abstract.

Wachowius, U., Talley, M., Silver, N., Heinze, H-J. & Sailer, M. (2005). Cognitive impairment in primary and secondary progressive multiple sclerosis, *Journal of Clinical and Experimental Neuropsychology, 27,* 65 – 77.

Ware, J. & Sherbourne, C. (1992). The MOS 36 – item short form health survey (SF-36). I. Conceptual framework and item selection. *Medical Care, 30*, 437 – 483.

Zivadinov, R., De Masi, R., Nasueli, D. Bragadin, L.M., Ukmar, M., Pozzi – Mucelli, R.S., Grop, A., Cazzato, G. & Zorzon, M. (2001). MRI techniques and cognitive impairment in the early phase of relapsing – remitting multiple sclerosis. *Neuroradiology, 43*, 272 – 278.

Zivadinov, R., Sepcic, J., Nasuelli, D., De Masi, R., Bragadin, L.M., Tommasi, M.A., Zambito – Marsala, S., Moretti, R., Bratince, A., Ukmar, M., Pozzi – Mucelli, R.S., Grop, A.,

Cazzato, G. & Zarzon, M. (2001). A longitudinal study of brain atrophy and cognitive disturbances in the early phase of relapsing – remitting multiple sclerosis. *Journal of Neurology, Neurosurgery, and Psychiatry, 70, 77*

INDEX

B

C

D

E

F

G

N

O

P

Q

R

S

T

U

V

W

X

Y